YOGA
FOR YOUR PERSONAL
FINANCES

Practical & Spiritual Solutions for Financial Health

Jacqueline Richards

Yoga for Your Personal Finances

© 2006 Jacqueline J. Richards

Jacqueline J. Richards
250 Greenbank Road, 8B Suite 124
Ottawa, ON K2H 1E9
www.jacquelinerichards.com
613-224-2982

Published by Book Coach Press
Ottawa, Ontario, Canada
www.BookCoachPress.com
info@BookCoachPress.com

Printed and bound in Canada

The advice and recommendations in this book are the opinion of the author and should in no way replace the services of qualified finance and health professionals. The author and publisher accept no responsibility for any injury that may result from attempting the yoga postures described in this book. If you have any health concerns, please consult your personal physician. Care has been taken to appropriately reference any books or quotations used in the writing of this book. The author and publisher welcome any information enabling them to rectify any references or credit in subsequent editions.

Production Manager: Serena Williamson
Editor: Karen Lanouette
Designer: Donald Lanouette
Printer: Tri-Co Group

Library and Archives Canada Cataloguing in Publication
Richards, Jacqueline J., 1967-
    Yoga for your personal finances / Jacqueline J. Richards.

ISBN 0-9739071-7-7
    1. Finance, Personal. 2. Health. 3. Hatha yoga. I. Title.
    HG179.R5158 2006   332.024   C2006-905080-5

Table Of Contents

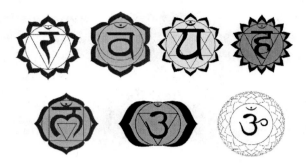

Introduction

*Expect your every need to be met, expect the answer to every problem,
expect abundance on every level, expect to grow spiritually.*

Eileen Caddy

Imagine sitting by the edge of a beautiful lake. Motionless and serene, you listen to the soothing sounds of the waves' ebb and flow. Your stillness has enticed a crimson dragonfly to perch on your bare shoulder. You watch the hawks soar overhead as the breeze brings you the scented pleasures of cedar. You are grateful for this moment in life.

As you leave this experience, you venture back to your personal reality, contemplating which bills will need to be paid on your return. Can you find a way to lend your sister a few dollars to ease some of the tension in her life? If the oil change is done in two weeks, instead of tomorrow, will this cause the engine to seize? Do you have the equipment ready for the next season of midget hockey, which starts next month? You forgot to do your business month-end report. Better work on that today.

You wonder where that free, unbounded crimson dragonfly disappeared to. You sit in your living room and wonder, "What have I allowed to happen in my life?"

How have we allowed our lives to become so difficult? I remember promising myself, "I'll never live like this when I grow up" and, "I'll never want for anything and I won't have to work hard for it." What happened to "I'll never work for less than my worth" and, "If I don't like my boss, I'm out of here!" Are we futilely endeavoring to keep up with the Joneses or the Trumps? From the time they entered the world, we believed that our children would be the next Albert Einstein, Rosa Parks, Tiger Woods or Warren Buffet. What kind of pressure do those expectations put on a child (or a parent)?

Money can be the source of all evil, or it can hold great happiness and ultimate success—and everything outside, over, and under. Debt is a four-letter word that is nervously stored underneath the bed or in the corner of a closet. Money puts a roof over our heads, grows the savings, and helps plan for the unforeseen and the inevitable.

Ask yourself, "How out of balance am I?" And, "How do I bring myself into balance?" The reality is, if you are reading this book, your finances are probably a bit chaotic and you are looking for a way to healthily balance your relationship with money.

I work in the financial industry, helping clients realize their dream of owning a home. Sadly, I have to tell more than a few people that they aren't able to afford it. What has struck me, as I reviewed their finances, is the unbalanced emotional relationship common to those who have the most problems with money. And, even though I'm a financial professional, I also have an imperfect relationship with money. I sometimes struggle to balance my needs and my wants. I want to shrug my shoulders and buy those amazing shoes with the money that's supposed to be paying my hydro bill.

I'm also a teacher and an ongoing student of yoga. I originally turned to yoga as a means of physical exercise, but became quickly aware of the emotional and mental benefits. I came to treasure that calm, reflective time as I worked through the *asanas* (postures). At the end of each class I was better able to deal with life's challenges. The more time I gave to yoga, the more balanced all aspects of my life became. I found that I had the inner resources to deal with the problems that had caused me so much distress—money, family and work. I hope that by sharing some of my insights as to how yoga can help you create a healthy relationship with money, you will find yourself living the comfortable, secure life you've always dreamed of. If you practice the actions suggested in each section, you will balance the satisfaction of meeting the needs of you and your family, along with some of the pleasures that having extra money can provide.

Yoga is considered a philosophy, a science and an art. Unknowingly, we practice yoga every day. Yoga is our group fitness class, our recreational sports, our stretching and bodybuilding. Our children practice yoga just by sitting on the floor in a kindergarten class. We practice yoga when we step outside of our office to catch a breath of air, or while sitting cross-legged at our firm's boardroom table.

Yoga has filtered into western society from India over the past hundred years. The earliest records of Yoga go back more than two thousand years. This centuries-old practice brings the body, mind, and spirit into harmony, uncluttered by the use of western medications, psychologists or psychoanalysts.

The word "yoga" means "union." Yoga is a form of exercise based on the belief that the body and breath are intimately connected with the mind. The concepts and techniques of yoga seek harmony between the material, mental and spiritual. Unmanageable finances are one manifestation of what happens when these three areas are out of balance. The stress you feel when you have an unhealthy relationship with money carries over into all aspects of your life, preventing any sense of joy or completion.

Aside from deep breathing and the often seen pretzel-like poses, the major piece of the yogic puzzle is the energy system known as the chakras.

Chakras are defined as a "wheel" of energy circuits. They are the juncture of life energy. There are seven major chakras, all connected to the essence of being that animates the human spirit.

These chakras are named: *Muladhara* (Root), *Svadhisthana* (Sacral), *Manipura* (Solar Plexus), *Anahata* (Heart), *Vissudha* (Throat), *Ajna* (Brow), and *Sahasrara* (Crown). Associated with the energies of these chakras are the physical poses, or *asanas*. When these chakras are out of balance, so is your life. When you use yoga to harmonize your energy circuits, you gain the physical and mental strength needed to take the steps that lead to healthy finances.

Take a moment to think about and then write down what your definition of healthy means, in terms of money. It will differ for each person, according to age, personal relationships and wants.

Survival needs are fairly basic—anywhere from 1800 to 3000 balanced calories a day and shelter that's appropriate for your environment. But what does *your* shelter need to be, in order to meet other needs that are based in emotions? Are you happy to rent a bachelor apartment, while saving to go travelling or amassing a down payment for a future home? Do you need at least four bedrooms and two bathrooms for your growing family? Are you able to pay your utility bills on time, or are you always getting those little red notices that threaten you with the loss of service? Do you always shop and cook for yourself, or do you dine out at the finest restaurants while hoping that your credit card won't be rejected? Are you able to afford that winter coat? Conversely, do you create chaos by buying a winter coat that isn't based on warmth, but on making sure that you have this season's look, worried that others will judge you, when, realistically, you can only afford about 20% of the coat's purchase price?

And so the years can go on, costing you the pleasures you could have bought if you took a bit of time to invest your money intelligently. Are you caught up in consumer mania? Does your friends' and family's "helpful" advice so overload you that you refuse to make a decision?

Write down the goals that you associate with financial health; perhaps some savings for emergencies and retirement, insurance to protect your family and possesions, no stress when paying the monthly bills, enough for a vacation every year, the ability to walk through your daily life knowing that you are in control of your finances rather than feeling at the mercy of them. Through the course of this book, you'll learn how to make these goals a reality.

The association of financial and money management practices, yoga, and the chakras may seem far-fetched in the 21st century. But it overlaps yogic beliefs that are centuries old.

It has been remarked that money keeps our societal score. If it didn't, you wouldn't see so many designer-name handbag knock-offs. Most of our games use terminology and rules for just that, score keeping. You will find evidence in this book to make you think twice about if you want to keep playing by the monetary scorecard and rulebook. At the very least, it will have you think about your past, current and future circumstances.

You may find that you do not have a perfect set, match, and game score with all three of these facets. If this is the case, you are in a position of imbalance. Your true self needs to shine through for a healthily balanced life.

Use these seven chapters to examine your beliefs about your money predicament, realign your misdirections, create your future goals for financial flexibility and freedom, and initiate the actions that will make them a reality.

Enjoy your journey through the seven chakras as you create a set of balanced, healthy financial attitudes.

Namaste,

Jacqueline

Your Chakra Balance Score Sheet

Begin your fundamental awareness of your finances and their functionality right now. Fill out the scorecard below Write first through your own eyes, and then through the eyes of your family and friends as to how they would gage you. Now, evaluate yourself through the eyes of who or what you deem to be your spiritual higher power.

Each question on the worksheet is a tool that will help you to understand how true you are to your own sense of self. Without this understanding, it is very difficult to have a healthy relationship with your finances. What do these three relationship zones say about your money management, your physical health and stress management, and your kindness quotient?

Assign a value of 0 to 5, where 0 is **no comment**, 1 is **extremely negative**, 2 **restrained**, 3 **supportive**, 4 **positive**, and 5 is **exceptionally optimistic**.

Chakra Balance	You	Friends & Family	Universe/ Spiritual Sources
Stable and predictable (Root Chakra)	4	3	2
Always fun-loving and in good spirits (Sacral Chakra)	4	5	5
Walking with strength and confidence (Solar Plexus Chakra)	5	5	5
Open to forgiving and choosing to forget (Heart Chakra)	4	3	3
Speaking with respect and diplomacy to others (Throat Chakra)	4	3	3
Trusting your gut instinct (Brow Chakra)	3	3	3
Always expressing thanks (Crown Chakra)	5	5	5
	29	27	26

What your scores mean

Under 42

You need to reposition from a sense of "lack" to the knowing that you can accomplish more. This book will help guide you on the path to success.

43 to 62

Practice being happy and appreciative every day for all that you have and all that is coming to you!

63 to 82

Appreciate your unique contributions to people's lives, including your own. Others appreciate you. Your journey of the mind, body and spirit is in place now and continues to facilitate your health and wealth.

Over 83

You are well on your way to self-enlightenment. Share your techniques and offer help to someone who is searching for guidance.

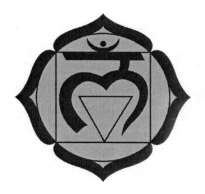

1ˢᵀ CHAKRA

Muladhara (Root)

I Am

Asanas (positions): Mountain & Yoga Squat

The *Muladhara* (Root) Chakra is the first energy system in the life wheel. If this chakra is balanced, you understand exactly what your needs are and have the confidence that you will meet them.

When you were born, your new environment was loud and confusing. For the first time you experienced hunger and cold. You needed food. Your mother's soothing, familiar voice and the warmth of her arms comforted you.

It can be devastating if these needs, basic to all infants, are not met. It manifests in adult life as an ongoing imbalance in the root chakra, meaning that you may never meet your basic requirements for shelter, human warmth and emotional security. Your inner voice will discouragingly chant "I can't" rather than the joyous "I can." You will recklessly fulfill wants, rather than take care of the essentials.

If you find yourself buying that expensive suit with the money you need to buy groceries and pay the hydro bill, your root chakra is out of balance. The high you got from shopping will quickly swing into guilty worry when you get the cut-off notice from the utility company. These negative feelings will unbalance you further, resulting in more unhealthy behaviours.

A balanced Root chakra will give you the energy and mental strength to reach your material goals. When balanced, there is equilibrium between the basic necessities for preservation of life.

The Conversation

This afternoon I had a conversation with a charming lady about her family vacation. It was a last-minute travel adventure, to take advantage of some family time during the March break. She had many friends who took chances booking last-minute vacations and they had always had a great time.

The question of whether or not they should take this trip reared its ugly head many times while Melonie was making the arrangements. Her employer was laying off 20% of the staff, and she was in the possible "pink slip" zone. Understandably, she felt that she needed a break. Melonie, despite her in-laws' cautions, chose to be spontaneous and live on the edge. Her husband is a "go for it" kind of guy. Funds and time were scarce, but…why not? Life is short!

She had some room on her credit cards. With the last-minute flights and insurance charged on the joint credit cards, she giggled to herself privately, "The cards haven't exploded yet! I'll get our budgeting back on track when we return. We can stay with friends and we won't need much more than a bit of money for food and some souvenirs. "

One week prior to the family's departure, she finally connected with her friends in London. Unfortunately, her friends were going to be in France. They, too, were taking advantage of some family time.

Melonie was still positive that she could get her family off on their vacation. She was determined to help her family enjoy the basics of life, no matter how stressful it currently was. She felt that the togetherness of the family supporting each other during a travel escape would be worth it. They had all been feeling alone, battling school exams and employment dilemmas.

Okay. Flight tickets were booked. She still needed a place to stay. Then she thought of her friend who had a vacation ownership package. It took three days but, for a price, he was able to book a place to stay. They were to leave in four days.

Melonie relaxed that evening, thinking that the worst had come and gone. That was when her youngest daughter started vomiting. Not once, not twice, but three times. She brought her daughter to the doctor, who confirmed, "It's just a little bug. She has the flu and will feel better in a few days."

With what felt like a thousand obstacles overcome, Melonie's family was packed and ready to head out on their adventure.

On the morning of their departure, Melonie woke up with a fever probably brought on by the huge stresses of trying to forceably create, an unplanned and unaffordable vacation. She didn't take care of the basics; she clearly didn't have the money, her credit card was maxed-out and her employment position was precarious. Melonie was not ensuring that her family's basic, root needs were being met. Melonie needed a budget.

The Money: My Budget Is In My Head

Happiness is not just something ready made.
It comes from your own actions.

The Dalai Lama

A Money Budget is the beginning of everything. What do you consider the basics? Housing, food, clothing, and utilities are obvious choices. But we also have other costs that are part of our comfort zone; the morning coffee, monthly manicures, entertainment, gym fees and so forth.

If you find yourself wanting to stand in the middle of the street and scream "Someone save me. Life's not fair and I want out!" then you are living in the stress brought on by your inability to meet basic needs.

Do you have a budget, a real and usable budget that tells you how much you spent on coffee at Tim Horton's, a budget that you check on a daily and weekly basis? If you don't, relax. Creating and sticking to a budget is not easy, but it is absolutely possible.

Building a budget will help overcome the unconscious behaviours and attitudes that keep your financial life in a constant state of disorder.

The following budget worksheet takes away the mystery. Set aside an hour, then sit down with this worksheet and think carefully about where you spend your money. Start filling in the blanks. Include items such as morning coffee, lunch breaks, movies, gas, and daycare, as well as the more obvious ones like rent/mortgage, groceries and utilities. Modify any payments that do not occur each month by adjusting them to represent a monthly payment.

Budget Worksheet

CATEGORY	BUDGET AMOUNT	ACTUAL AMOUNT	DIFFERENCE
REVENUES/INCOME			
Wages and Bonuses			
Miscellaneous Income			
Income Subtotal			
Less the following taxes			
Federal/Provincial			
Income Tax			
Other Taxes			
MONTHLY EXPENSES			
HOME			
Mortgage or Rent			
Homeowners/ Renters Insurance			
Property Taxes			
Home Repairs/Maintenance/ Condominium Fees			
Home Improvements			
UTILITIES			
Electricity			
Water and Sewer			
Natural Gas or Oil			
Telephone (Land Line, Cell)			

CATEGORY	BUDGET AMOUNT	ACTUAL AMOUNT	DIFFERENCE
FOOD			
Groceries			
Eating Out, Lunches, Snacks			
FAMILY OBLIGATIONS			
Child Support/Alimony			
Day Care, Babysitting			
HEALTH AND MEDICAL			
Insurance (Medical, Dental, Vision)			
Out-of-Pocket Medical Expenses			
Fitness (Yoga, Massage, Gym)			
TRANSPORTATION			
Car Payments			
Gasoline/Oil			
Auto Repairs/Maintenance/Fees			
Auto Insurance			
Other (Bus, Train, Subway, Taxi)			
DEBT PAYMENTS			
Credit Cards			
Student Loans			
Other Loans			
ENTERTAINMENT/RECREATION			
Cable TV/Videos/Movies			
Computer Expenses			
Hobbies			
Subscriptions and Dues			
Vacations			
PETS			
Food			
Grooming, Boarding, Vet			
CLOTHING			
INVESTMENTS AND SAVINGS			
RRSP, RESP			
Stocks/Bonds/Mutual Funds			
Savings			
Emergency Fund			
MISCELLANEOUS			
Toiletries, Household Goods			
Gifts/Charitable Donations			
Grooming (Hair, Make-up, Other)			
Miscellaneous Expense			
Total Monthly Investments & Expenses			
Surplus/Shortage (Monthly spending income minus expenses & investments)			

Setting Goals

Now that you have a picture of your financial situation, it's time for the actions that lead to financial health.

Complete the following goal worksheet. If you have a spouse, I suggest you first do this by yourself and then sit down with your partner and fill it in together.

Choose three small goals that you can attain within a month's time. As you take steps to accomplish each of these goals, celebrate. Pat yourself on the back and continue to be inspired.

Sample goals

· I begin to feel financially secure when I pay more than the minimum payment on my credit card.

· I begin to feel financially secure when I switch from an extra-large coffee to a large, saving myself $20 per month.

· I begin to feel financially secure when I meet a friend for tea, instead of a restaurant meal that I can't afford.

Now, fill in at least three of your own goals

I begin to feel financially secure when:

I pack a lunch

I begin to feel financially secure when:

I use the money in my pocket not
on my cards.

I begin to feel financially secure when:

I see commission checks and my paypal account fill up with money.

Feel free to set new goals once you feel you've got a handle on the ones you've just set down. As you become more practiced in money management, you can start setting more ambitious goals.

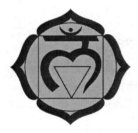

The Asanas: Mountain & Yoga Squat

Practicing these asanas will align your energy and enhance the physical and mental stability needed to begin and maintain the tasks that lead to financial health.

Posture : *Tadasana* (Mountain)

The Sanskrit word *tada* means mountain. This posture is also known by the name *samasthiti-asana*. *Sama* means unmoved and *sthiti* means standing upright. Combined, *samasthiti* means standing firmly without moving.

- Stand with ankles close together, breathe gently.

- Feel a lengthening in the entire body.

- While your big toes are pressing together and your legs are also pressing together, bring the belly to the spine.

- Soften your knees and relax the shoulders.

Tadasana (Mountain)

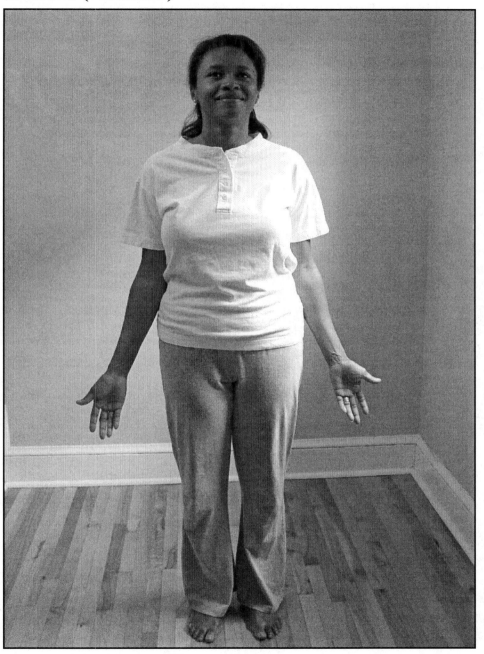

Posture: *Utkatasana* (Chair Pose or Yoga Squat)

Utkata means powerful. The Yoga Squat works the muscles of the arms and legs, and also stimulates the diaphragm and heart.

- Start in the Mountain posture.

- Inhale while stretching your arms overhead.

- Put arms in prayer position.

- Exhaling, bend in toward your knees, heels anchored into the ground.

- Your abs should be pulled in and your torso slightly forward.

Utkatasana (Chair Pose or Yoga Squat)

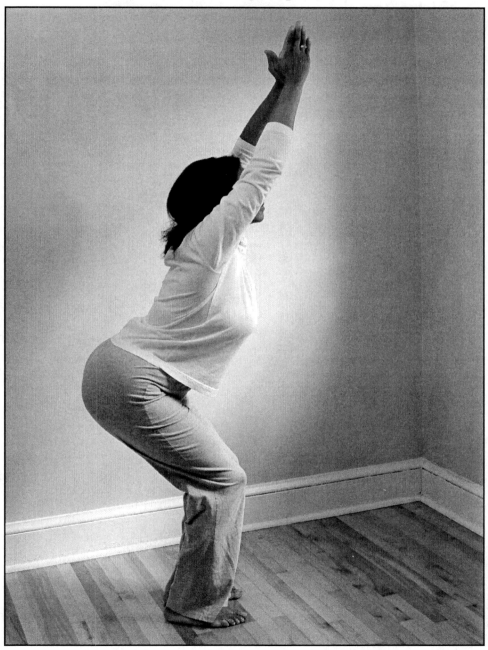

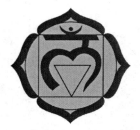

1st Chakra: Additional Information

- The gemstone specific to this chakra is carnelian.
- The associated essential oils are jojoba and patchouli.
- Red is the primary colour for this chakra.
- The sound mantra for meditation is "Lam."
- The sense associated with this chakra is smell.
- The Muladhara (Root) chakra is located at the base of the spine and opening of the anus.
- The challenge of "I am" is to find a balance between your need for rigid control and your urge to totally give in to life's currents.
- The element associated with this chakra is Earth. The journey toward the balanced life you seek begins when you apply the grounded energy of this chakra to your finances.

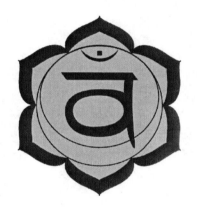

2ND CHAKRA

Svadhisthana   (Sacral/Navel)

I Feel

Asanas (positions): Child & Cow-face

The *Svadhisthana* (Sacral) Chakra is the second energy system in the life wheel. It is the location of sensuality and the appetite for life's pleasures. When this chakra is in balance you experience the material world as both healthy and pleasurable. You walk fearlessly, enjoying a sense of curiosity.

Anger, pain, guilt, and shame are all results of the disturbance of the positive flow within the Sacral chakra. When this chakra is unbalanced, you resist change. You reject the positive information of your senses and miserably isolate yourself from friends and family. You may find yourself spending wildly in an attempt to feel better, only to sink further into depression when the bills come due.

In this chapter you will learn how rebalance this chakra and move on. You will even feel gratitude for having learned a thing or two from your mistakes. When your Sacral chakra is balanced, your inner voice proclaims, "I will create my life, and I will create a future filled with abundance. I'm going to use all of the resources that I have to create this future."

The Conversation

They were latchkey kids. They were taught that a messy room meant a messy life. When the alarm clock bell sounded, they got up immediately and made their beds. There was no chatting about the reasons they didn't buy Count Chocula cereal—they understood they were lucky to have the extra-large bag of Puffed Wheat. Amelia, the oldest, sprinkled enough sugar on her Puffed Wheat that it layered the bottom of her bowl when the cereal was finished. Then she would scoop up her leftover milk and the sugar granules; it was her morning treat.

Amelia made everyone's lunch. They had enough bologna or processed cheese for sandwiches, but never enough for bologna and cheese sandwiches. For a snack, they had one Wagon Wheel or three chocolate chip cookies, but not the Wagon Wheel and chocolate chip cookies. The children dressed for school and left the house, carefully locking the door with the key that Amelia kept around her neck.

In school, Amelia shifted, becoming the class rebel, chewing prohibited gum and socializing during a much-needed class education. This conduct got her moved to an empty corner in the back of the classroom. That was okay, as she could daydream about the dreamiest Grade Five teacher in the universe, and it would never matter to him if she passed his class. Just so long as she was happy.

When the bell rang, signifying that the school day was done, Amelia walked back with her girlfriends, giggling about the day's events before arriving home. She then switched back to the dutiful daughter, the oldest of three, as she made sure that the other kids did their homework and chores until Mom got home from work.

It's the way it was. Amelia's mom, like many single parents in her position, worked hard to provide opportunities for her children. She hoped to give them the magical options that she herself never had. She knew she was giving them responsibilities greater than their peers', she knew she was missing so much of their lives, but she had no choice.

Now grown into an imaginative and savvy businesswoman, Amelia began by painting and selling unique T-shirts that spoke of the unique experiences found in various professions. She expanded her market into painting artistic handcrafted signs and items for small and medium businesses, and she has done well while indulging her love of creative expression.

One problem. As Amelia travels coast-to-coast with her wares, she hopes for the ability to consistently pay the bills. Sometimes the payments are on time, and sometimes they are close to being on time. She'd better check the hydro payment. Amelia does not enjoy the phone calls to negotiate the electricity bill. She needs power to run the sewing machine and silkscreen operation. She is dreaming about a factory that she could call her own. But it is just that, a dream.

She had better make time to assess her financial state to ensure that she is on her game. She may not know it, but the credit bureaus and potential lending institutions have already measured her. Amelia worked hard to get the key to the front door, but how will she unlock it?

The Money: Credit Past, Present and Future

Bad habits are like chains that are too light to feel
until they are too heavy to carry.
Warren Buffett

There are three sides to a financial record; your story, the banks and credit card companies' story, and the record that the credit bureaus keep of your spending.

To understand your financial situation you will need to evaluate your previous financial behaviour, your current circumstances and your anticipated future.

The budget you created in the last chapter gave you a snapshot of your current situation. Now, let's unlock the mystery of credit. You need to know the purpose of credit bureaus, how your credit is reported and then evaluated, and how to avoid the increasingly common phenomena of identification fraud.

Your Credit Past

The credit bureaus have the task of gathering your financial information and giving any potential moneylender your money management history. You may be as young as sixteen when they start tracking your borrowing and spending habits. In this context, when we talk about money management, it begins with your first credit application.

Did you take out a student loan to help with college or university? Did you remember to pay that loan back? I can tell you that the Canadian Student Loan Corporation did not forget. After many, many attempts at contacting you, they sent your file to a collections agency, which notified the credit bureaus that you were delinquent on your loan payment.

A credit report tracks how consistently you pay your financial obligations. If you have borrowed money from credit card companies, department stores and banks, they regularly inform the credit bureaus about the length of time you have been involved with the company, whether you make your payments on time, if you miss a payment, or if you have gone over your credit limit.

The credit bureaus are financial "big brothers," seeing everything we have done; good, bad or ugly. Lenders use the information to decide whether to grant you credit or a loan. Your credit report is the history they use to determine what kind of lending risk you are.

If you are starting to despair, have hope. You can build a better credit rating. Even bankruptcies are taken off your credit record after seven years.

Your Current Credit

You can find out your credit score by contacting either Equifax Canada (www.equifax.ca) or TransUnion (www.transunion.com).

Your credit score determines your credit worthiness. The higher the score, the better you are as a risk. Your credit score will also help determine the interest rate you pay on your loan or credit card.

If your score is

720 or above
Financial institutions should provide a quick acceptance for your request.

620 to 720
They will take a closer look at your file. The lender may ask you to explain the bureaus' reports with any mitigating factors.

Less than 620
It may take a little bit of time to find suitable financing. Interest rates may be higher because you represent a higher risk category.

Reasons for your score

- You have past delinquencies on more than one account.
- You are carrying balances and only making minimum payments.
- You have limited credit lines to judge credit worthiness by.
- You have looked for and have often been denied credit.
- You changed employers frequently.
- You have moved many times.
- Your reported income does not support your debt-load.

Your Credit Future

Once they understand the meaning of credit reports and score, many of my clients ask what can they do to improve their credit score. I suggest three things that will quickly improve credit rating.

1. Pay all of your bills on time. Late payments have a negative impact on your score.

2. Stay well within 75% of the available limits of your credit cards and overdraft.

3. Do not apply for multiple credit cards. Unless you need the card, don't get it. With each application, your bureau file will be accessed, negatively impacting your credit rating.

If you know that you have impacted your credit rating due to an explainable circumstance (a few months of unpaid bills due to a critical illness, for example), you can request in writing that the credit bureaus document this reason in your records.

In order to bring your finances into balance, you need to become more conscious of how you use credit. Just as yoga balances your chakras and unifies body and mind, the quick credit card evaluation below gives you a tool to determine whether your credit costs are out of alignment.

You may be paying for service charges that are unnecessary. Do you really need to pay that extra interest on your Air Miles card if you haven't taken a trip in three years?

Quick Credit Card Evaluation

· Do you have ATM access for cash advances on your credit card? If so, do you start to pay interest as soon as you take out a cash advance or do you get an interest-free period during which you can make a payment?

· Are you charged annual service fees?

· Do you have a free Air Miles or a Rewards program, or do you pay a premium on these programs?

· Do you have protection against loss, theft, or ID fraud? If so, do you use your card in risky enough situations to warrant the fees?

· Do you have low introductory interest rates? If so, will you be able to keep your balance at zero when the high interest rates kick in?

Review your answers, check the fees or extra interest involved versus the benefits, and determine if you need to contact the lender to make changes that will save you money.

ID Fraud

Identity theft is more than just someone stealing your credit card number. Using basic personal information like name, address and social insurance number, identity thieves open credit card accounts, lease or buy cars, rent apartments, and buy electronic goods and jewelry, using the stolen name.

You can limit the potential for fraud by remembering a few key tips.

· Carry only the identification and credit cards you need when travelling, whether locally or abroad.

· Never leave your purse or wallet unattended. Keep your personal data and information guarded at all times.

· If your statements stop arriving, contact your bank. Read through your monthly statements carefully.

· When making a purchase, keep your cards in view at all times; ensure that you take your card back as soon as a transaction swipe has been completed with your card.

· Always save your receipts, never leave them behind. Do not sign a blank charge slip.

· Avoid saying your account number aloud so that others can hear.

· Only provide your ID and credit card information over the phone to reputable companies with whom you have initiated the call.

· If you receive a call from someone claiming to represent your credit card issuer and the caller asks for your account number, do not provide it. If the issuer employs the caller, they will already know your account information.

· If your Social Insurance Card is lost or stolen, contact your employer or your local Human Resources Development (HRDC) office immediately.

· If your Driver's License is lost or stolen, contact your local driver and vehicle license issuing office and report it to your local police station.

· Make a list of the names, account numbers and expiration dates of all your cards and store it in a safe place (separate from your cards). This will come in handy if you must alert credit issuers about a lost or stolen card.

· Call all of your credit issuers immediately upon discovering that your cards are missing. Most have 24-hour service numbers for this purpose. If you re-open the account, ensure they have your correct personal information.

Despite your best efforts, it's possible you could become a victim of identity theft or credit card fraud. If you suspect you are a victim, you should immediately:

· Call your bank/financial institution.

· Call the local police and ask for the fraud squad, if they have one.

· Call Phonebusters at 1-877-495-8501 or www.phonebusters.com for telemarketing fraud.

· Place a "Fraud Alert" on your credit bureaus; Equifax at 1-800-465-7166 or www.equifax.ca. TransUnion at 1-866-525-0262 or www.tuc.ca.

· Check your financial statements carefully for three to six months to make sure that the problem has been completely resolved.

Creating your new, healthy credit score will take some effort and vigilance. Sadly, it's much less fun than the shopping sprees that might explain why your rating is unsatisfactory. But if your *Svadhisthana* (Sacral) chakra is in balance, you will find it easier to work at improving your credit rating.

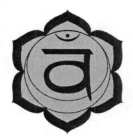

The Asanas: Child & Cow-face

Practicing these *asanas* will give you the ability to move easily and calmly with the fast-flowing currents of your life, preventing the stress that leads to unhealthy financial choices.

Posture: *Bala-asana* (Child)

The Sanskrit word *bala* means child. This pose mimics the fetal position in the womb. The entire spinal column is stretched, opening and calming the lumbar and nervous system.

- In kneeling position sit on your heels with toes pointed behind you.

- Separate knees to approximately hip width.

- Bend till forehead touches the floor, then place your arms with palms turned upward beside your torso.

- Modify this pose into the Diamond pose by positioning your arms forward on the floor.

Bala-asana (Child)

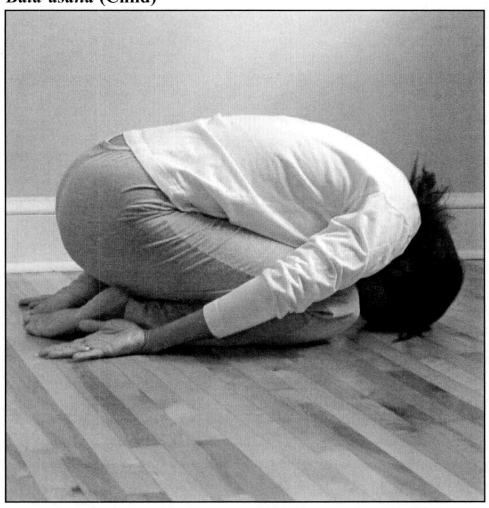

Posture: *Gomukhasana* (Cow-face)

Go means cow and *Mukha* means face. When viewed from behind this posture resembles the face of the cow. Also, *go* can mean light, so *gomukh* also refers to the light in or of the head.

- Sit on floor, cross your legs and relax hips and thighs to the side.
- Keep your back straight.
- Lower your right arm, bending it at the elbow, and raise your hand and forearm behind your back. Clasp your fingers so that you hook your hands together, or clasp your hands palm to palm.
- In either case, take care that your hands are centered in line with your spine and between your shoulder blades.
- Clasp hands firmly and keep hands and torso centered. Head and eyes look straight ahead.
- If you need it, use a strap to help connect your hands behind you.
- Reverse arms and repeat.

Gomukhasana (Cow-face)

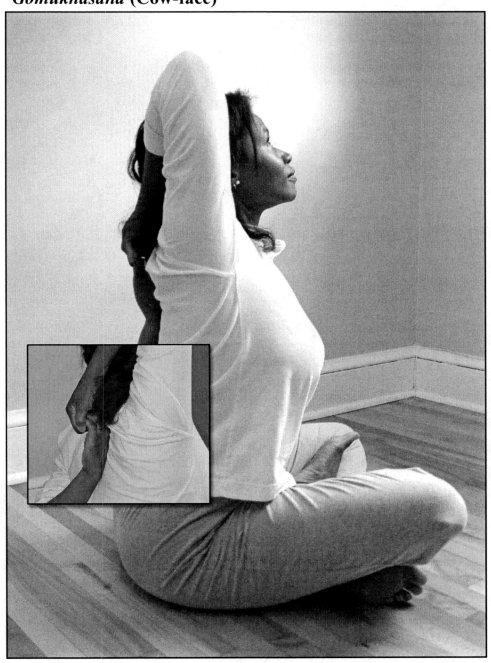

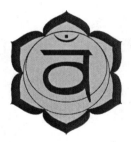

2nd Chakra: Additional Information

- The gemstone specific to this chakra is amber.
- The associated essential oils are lemon grass and orange.
- Orange is the primary colour for this chakra.
- The sound mantra for meditation is "Vam."
- The sense associated with this chakra is smell.
- The Sacral chakra is aptly named. It is located in the navel region.
- The challenge of "I feel" lies in understanding that you have the ability to enter, maintain, change or leave any relationship in your life.
- The element water represents the Sacral chakra. Our inner movements originate within the element of water. It is the never-ending ebb and flow of this element which manages our "fight or flight" reflexes. In this chapter, you will learn how to swim calmly through the waters of your financial state.

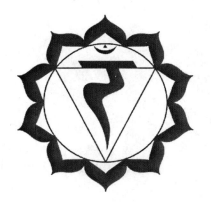

3ᴿᴰ CHAKRA

Manipura (Solar Plexus)
I Can
Asanas (positions): Camel & Boat

The third energy center in the life wheel is the *Manipura* (Solar Plexus) chakra. It is the location of both your sense of self and physical power. Balance in this chakra means a healthy sense of self-esteem that enables sensible risks as you claim power over your finances.

If this chakra is out of balance, you will suffer from low self-worth. This can show up as either co-dependent behaviour, handing over your power to others—all the while secretly resenting them—or as a rigid perfectionism in which no job is ever done well enough and no praise is high enough. Overspending in an attempt to bolster your self-esteem creates financial problems. Your money management is also impacted by the fact that you may have employment troubles due to problems created by your unbending attitudes or out-of-control people pleasing.

As you rebalance this chakra you will learn to accept and appreciate yourself for who you are, all the while knowing that you have the power to make changes for the better. You will no longer feel the need to manipulate others in order to feel good about yourself. You will find yourself being of service in the world, rather than suspiciously trying to make sure you get your fair share.

A balanced Solar Plexus chakra gives you the inner resources to change attitudes and habits that are barriers to your financial health.

The Conversation

We are products of our environment. We learn from early experiences and formal education. Sometimes the way is easy and sometimes there are barriers that seem impossible to surmount. We have to muster our confidence to confront the dangers to our self-worth. We protect our family, our friends, and ourselves.

Recently, my family enjoyed the blessing of a beautiful day at a cottage overlooking a lake. From the front porch we watched a large black crow circle the cottage and the calm lake waters. Was it looking for frogs, insects, a refuge, or something known only to the mind of a crow? It landed on the roof with a thud.

Immediately, a small swallow attacked the crow. We realized that this David and Goliath scene was because the swallow was protecting her nest. I worried that the swallow would lose her life fighting for the new babies she had so recently brought into this passionate world. These young swallows might lose their mother, and the power and experience she would pass on to her young. The mother had to succeed in this struggle so that her chicks would survive. A final dive bomb from the mother sent the crow into retreat.

It must have been a terrifying experience for the swallow. But, in the service of her young, she became a mighty warrior. The tiny mother sparrow taught us a lesson. Do not give up against what seems like an unbeatable opponent—whether a crow or your hemorrhaging cash flow and debt crisis. You can become a financial warrior to protect yourself and your loved ones.

This is where you take action. Make the decision that now is not too late! You're twice as likely to be struck by lightning as win the lottery, so it's time to make some small changes that will give you the power to begin investing.

The Money: Take Hold of Your Financial Power Plan

The richest soil, if uncultivated, produces the rankest weeds.

Plutarch

It is never too late to have a strategy. With careful preparation you will use your money to make more money. Investing your hard-earned money should never become a risk or a gamble.

As you take control of your financial situation, know that it is not dishonest, dishonourable, or unattractive to be rich. It simply puts more power into your hands.

Read some basic books on investing. Attend some of the free workshops and seminars that are offered in your areas, but take away only information, not a contract to buy their stocks. Book an appointment with a financial professional.

These strategies will help to take away your fear of money, and to calm those inner voices that may claim you don't deserve wealth, or tell you you couldn't manage money if you did have it.

Five Building Blocks On the Road to Financial Freedom

Wealth building is a result of organization, planning, and motivation. Take these five tips to heart in your plans to be financially independent.

1. Congratulate yourself for taking control and beginning to build your personal wealth. As in the first chapter, set a goal and then enjoy creating the strategy to achieve it. The hardest part is to commit to your goals. Keep your goal fires burning.

2. When you save and invest a portion of your income, you begin to reap the benefits of your money at work. We'll talk about the miracle of compound interest further on.

3. Live within your means and make sure that saving five to ten percent of your monthly income is part of your plan.

4. Always pay yourself first (i.e. save), by putting a little extra away for rainy day emergencies. Then systematically pay out the higher interest debts.

5. Envision the field of wealth and ride toward it, *now*. Any amount contributed to your savings, no matter how small, is significant. And when it is time, bring in a trusted financial advisor to review your unique scenario.

In the previous chapters you met Melonie and Amelia. If Melonie had created financial goals that included her family vacation, she would have avoided some of the mayhem that took place. With enough funds in place to pre-book the vacation and compensate for her time (regardless of her employment issues) she could have gone on her vacation with peace of mind, knowing that she wasn't creating future financial havoc for her family.

Amelia used her creative gifts to create a viable enterprise, but constantly juggles the basic funds needed to operate it. Her upbringing has provided her with the inner resources to expand her business, but she must remember to balance her spending to support all her business needs. Amelia needs the money to make sure that the operation continues to run with the lights on.

Both of these clients need to take charge of fine-tuning their finances. Using compounding interest is one of the best ways of achieving that goal. Start today by simply taking a dollar a day out of your coffee or gum habit. If you were to put that dollar into the bank every day for the next ten years and then leave it untouched for another ten, the miracle of compound interest would turn it into almost $20,000 by the end of twenty years.

Creating a plan for financial success

Compounding means that you earn interest on both your principal and interest. You'll have to put your money into long-term investments, but the results are worth it.

Strategize with the *Rule of 72* and plan your victory. You can quickly calculate how long it will take to double your money based on the interest rate your investment averages.

Here's how it works

Divide 72 by the interest rate you expect to earn. This will show the number of years it will take to double your money. For example, if your investment fund earns 8% interest, use this formula this way:

The magical number	Divided by the interest rate	Equals the number of years
72	8%	9 years

The chart on the following page shows the impact of saving just one dollar a day over a full year. If you continued this saving's plan for twenty years, you would contribute $7,170 of your own money and you would earn $17,788 in interest (based on a 10% average annual return rate).

Your Buck a Day Worksheet

	Sample Savings at $30.00/month at 10% interest	Sample Challenges and Successes		Savings at $30.00/month at ___ % interest	My Challenges and Successes
Month No. 0	$ 30.00	One year to go of saving one coffee (out of my 5 coffees) a day!	My Month No. 0	$	
Month No. 1	$ 30.00 plus $30 plus 0.25 interest = $60.25	I think my body is thanking me for one less coffee! And my boss is, too...	My Month No. 1		
Month No. 2	$ 60.25 plus $30 plus 0.50 interest = $90.75	Okay, I splurged and bought a designer coffee. But I put the money back in!	My Month No. 2	$	
Month No. 3	$ 90.75 plus $30 plus 0.76 interest = $121.51	I'm trying to stay on track	My Month No. 3	$	
Month No. 4	$121.51 plus $30 plus 1.02 interest =$152.53		My Month No. 4	$	
Month No. 5	$152.53 plus $30 plus 1.28 interest =$183.81	I thought I couldn't save a dime!	My Month No. 5	$	
Month No. 6	$183.81 plus $30 plus 1.54 interest =$215.35	I am a Financial Warrior in training.	My Month No. 6	$	
Month No. 7	$215.35 plus $30 plus 1.80 interest =$247.15	Okay, I splurged and bought a coffee maker to make my own designer coffee. And I put the money back in.	My Month No. 7	$	
Month No. 8	$247.15 plus $30 plus 2.07 interest = $279.22		My Month No. 8	$	
Month No. 9	$279.22 plus $30 plus 2.34 interest = $311.56	It's not so complicated!	My Month No.9	$	
Month No. 10	$311.56 plus $30 plus 2.61 interest = $344.17		My Month No. 10	$	
Month No. 11	$344.17 plus $30 plus 2.88 interest = $377.05		My Month No. 11	$	
Month No. 12	$377.05 plus $30 plus 2.88 interest = $409.93	I am a Financial Warrior and I Invest!	My Month No. 12	$	

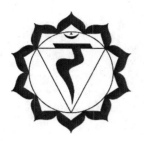

The *Asanas*: Camel & Boat

Practicing these asanas enhances your core strength and stamina, while increasing your flexibility. They help to provide the personal power that you will need to take charge of your financial health.

Posture: *Ushtra-asana* (Camel)

Ushtra is Sanskrit for camel. This animal survives in the desert by storing water in its body so it can use it when needed. Humans store knowledge which, when used appropriately, nourishes our spirits. The Camel pose revitalizes the mind.

- Sit up straight on your knees.
- Inhale and bend backwards, placing your right hand on your right heel.
- This is the half camel.
- Placing both hands on both heels completes a full camel.
- Remember to lift your chest up while dropping the head back.

Ushtra-asana (Camel)

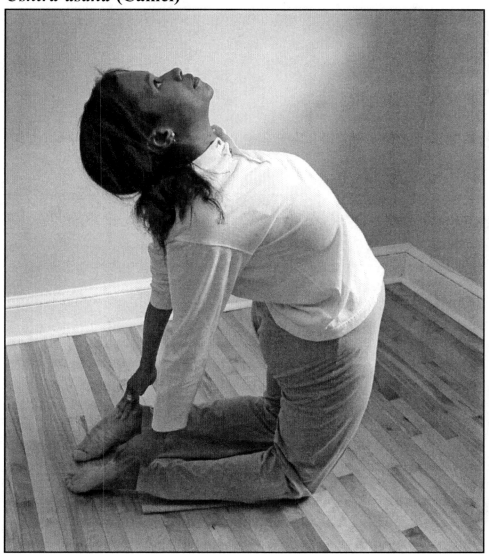

Posture: *Paripurna Navasana* (Boat Pose)

Pari is Sanskrit for full, or complete. *Nava* means boat. The Boat Pose a core strengthener for the vessel that is your body. Your "boat" can enjoyably take you anywhere, just as steering your financial boat becomes a pleasure, but unless your hull is in good repair, you won't get very far.

- Sit on the floor with your legs straight in front of you. Put hands behind hips, fingers pointed towards feet and press into the floor. Lengthen your torso and lean back slightly (don't let your back round).
- Bend your knees and lift your feet off the floor until your thighs are at a 45-degree angle. Straighten your knees until your toes are just above eye level. If this is too difficult, keep your knees bent but try to get your shins parallel to the floor.
- Stretch your arms alongside your legs and reach strongly out through your fingers. If this isn't possible, keep your hands on the floor beside your hips or hold on to the backs of your thighs.

Paripurna Navasana (**Boat Pose**)

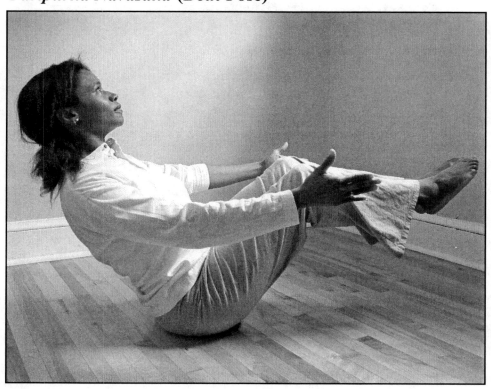

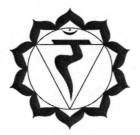

3RD Chakra: Additional Information

· The gemstone specific to this chakra is tiger's eye.

· The associated essential oils are bergamot and rosemary.

· Yellow is the primary colour for this chakra.

· The sound mantra for meditation is "Ram."

· The sense associated with this chakra is sight.

· The chakra is located in the abdominal and upper intestinal region.

· The challenge of "I can" is to remember that you have the power to choose what you think and how you behave.

· The element associated with this chakra is fire. It is the flame that feeds your courage and will to change. It is the warmth of your gratitude for all that is good in life. It is the source of the energy you need to implement financial changes.

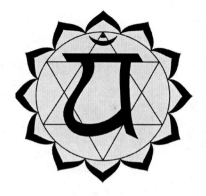

4ᵀᴴ CHAKRA

Anahata (Heart)

I Love

Asanas (positions): Half Spinal Twist & Crescent Moon

The *Anahata* (Heart) is the center point of the life wheel. It unifies the lower (physical) and higher (spiritual) energy circuits. Balance in the Heart chakra encourages tolerance of your and others' foibles.

In Sanskrit, *Anahata* translates as unhurt, meaning that, despite life's blows, your heart still holds wholeness, manifested in the will to love. When this chakra becomes unbalanced toward the intellect, you may find your judgmental behaviours push away your loved ones. Alternatively, when the *Anahata* is too open, over-empathy with others' anger or misery can plunge you into melancholy. You may lack the optimism necessary to make a comfortable home a financial priority.

Yoga helps integrate the upper and lower energy circuits of your body. If your Heart chakra is too open, rebalancing it enables you to slow down and take care of yourself before attending to others' needs. If the circuit is too closed, integration takes down your unnecessary defenses, opening you to the love that your family and friends have been trying to give all along.

Although we think of finances as governed by the head, the heart far more often controls them. As long as your heart is healthy, so are your finances. If your heart is governed by fear, it may manifest financially as either greed or the refusal to look at your debt-load because you doubt you have the resources to deal with the problems your unconscious spending habits have brought upon you

This chakra most applies to the financial health of your home, which is, after all, where the heart is. The loving welcome that every family member, friend and colleague who walks through your door should feel is far easier to manifest when your home's security is not in danger because of poor financial decisions—or lack of decisions.

The Conversation

I've had many conversations with clients and friends about home ownership. There are some responses that you can predict two time zones away. Others take you by surprise.

With the power of conviction, my Mom said, "Girl, husbands may come and husbands may go. But you bes' make sure you put a roof over your kids' heads!" Handed down from generation to generation, she believed this was a basic part of a parent's responsibility, an instinctive expression of love. My soon-to-be husband heard a similar sermon delivered from his "Enlightened One." His Mom said, "Son, a good woman who makes you happy is hard to find. But you bes' make sure you help her put a roof over your kids' heads!" I guess we are all on the same page.

The family is newly arrived in Canada. Mom and Dad made the decision that, for their children's sake, the stress of the mind, body and spirit generated by moving to a new country would be worth it. Mom and Dad each work two jobs over various shifts. This ensures that the kids always have a parent at home when they leave for school and when they return from a challenging day of learning. It also means that Mom and Dad only see each other for a shared family moment at dinner. Dad has just returned from work and now Mom leaves for her night shift. They are working so hard because they are saving for the down payment for a house. They used to have a home they called their own. Now they have an apartment they call the landlord's. But every month, by carefully managing their money, they are saving for the day they can purchase their own secure home.

She is seventy years old, a patient and giving mom, a playful and generous grandma, a loving and heartbroken widow, and a supportive friend with a fantastic belly laugh. She has just passed on the matriarch's torch to her children. Instead of hosting the Christmas dinner, Easter dinner, Surprise Anniversary parties, Birthday luncheons, and (with the grandchildren) Saturday pool parties, she now attends as the invited guest. She doesn't need the big house any more. Her friends have the most fantastic condominium apartments with a party room that hosts swing dancing lessons, and a hair salon. "I can have my hair done right there! Fancy that!" It is time to call a realtor and arrange the sale of her family home, despite the sorrow that she feels at losing the dwelling which holds her memories. The house she and her husband bought so many years ago will generate a profit that enables her to outright buy a physically manageable condo, plus bank some money for any future needs, and leave her grandchildren a nice inheritance.

For all of my clients, "Home is where the heart is."

The Money: Your Building Blocks

And hie him home, at evening's close, to sweet repast and calm repose.

Thomas Gray

Once you have made the decision that you intend to buy a home, it is time to look at the following four areas.

1. Credit

· Credit History.

· Credit Score.

· Client Character (employment stability, etc.).

All these factors will be considered in your mortgage application.

2. Down Payment Options

· Use your savings or up to $20,000 from your RRSP (if it's your first home).

· Use a gifted or borrowed down payment (usually from family).

· Use a Zero Down mortgage program (you will need about 2% of purchase price available in cash to meet the associated fees).

If your bank refuses to give you a mortgage, you may find that a mortgage broker has more leeway in granting you one.

3. Budgets & Goals

· Start with your comfort level. If you are renting for $850, a mortgage of $1,800 per month probably won't be a manageable payment.

· Lenders decide how big a mortgage you can afford using the Total Debt Ratio Service (TDS) and the Gross Debt Ratio Service (GDS) models (explained on page 56). Fill out the worksheets on the following pages to get an idea of the mortgage amount that you can afford.

· Set realistic home purchase expectations, whether it is your first or tenth purchase.

4. The Purchase

· Tour the areas that you want to live in. Check out the location's transport options, shopping, schools, libraries, cinemas, restaurants, etc.

· Create your team of experts. Find a mortgage expert, a real estate agent, a home inspector, and a lawyer to help you successfully and safely complete your purchase.

· Consider seeking a Pre-approved mortgage certificate. It means you can make an immediate offer (subject to confirmation of financing and home inspection, of course) when you find the right home.

Sample Mortgage Application

Below is a sample of a typical mortgage loan document. The Assets and Liabilities section on the next page gives you an idea of your net worth (it may reassure you to know that a small negative net worth is not always bad news).

Fill out this sample application to make sure that you have all the information available that your lender requires.

Applicant		Co-Applicant	
Date of birth:	SIN:	Date of birth:	SIN:
Marital status:	No. of dependents:	Marital status:	No. of dependents:
Current employer:		Current employer:	
Position:	Phone:	Position:	Phone:
Annual income: $	Yrs. of service:	Annual income: $	Yrs. of service:
Previous employer:		Previous employer:	
Position:		Position:	
Annual income: $	Yrs. of service:	Annual income: $	Yrs. of service:
Other income: $	Source:	Other income: $	Source:
Bank name:		Bank name:	
Bank address:		Bank address:	

Assets		Liabilities		Lender	Balance Owing	Monthly Payment
Value of home (if owned)	$	Mortgage(s) on home	1.		$	$
			2.		$	$
Cash in Bank	$	Personal loan(s)	1.		$	$
Deposit on purchase	$		2.		$	$
Other real estate owned	1. $	Other real estate loan(s)	1.		$	$
	2. $		2.		$	$
Cars	1. $	Car loan(s) or lease(s)	1.		$	$
	2. $		2.		$	$
RRSPs	$	Credit Cards	1.		$	$
Stocks, bonds, term deposits etc.	1. $		2.		$	$
	2. $		3.		$	$
Other	$		4.		$	$
	$	Child support/alimony			$	$
	$					
Total Assests	$	**Total Liabilities**			$	$

Now that you have completed your sample mortgage application, you can make a quick calculation to see how big a mortgage you can afford.

The Gross Debt Service (GDS) ratio represents the 32% of your gross income that is used to calculate your maximum mortgage. It includes things like property taxes, condominium fees, heating and, of course, your monthly mortgage payment.

If your household income per year is $72,000 (or $6,000 per month), your GDS ratio would be $23,040 (or $1,920/month).

The Total Debt Service (TDS) ratio includes the GDS plus household debt like credit cards, car payments or leases, student or personal loans, alimony and childcare payments. Regular expenses such as daycare, gas, groceries and insurance are not included. Your maximum TDS cannot be more than 40% of your income.

Back to the household income per year of $72,000 (or $6,000 per month); the maximum TDS ratio would be $28,800 (or 2,400/month).

Remember that the right lender may have leeway for your unique circumstances. Your dream of a home is very possible.

Gross and Total Debt Service Calculator

Read through the sample numbers and then enter your personal numbers to calculate the mortgage that you are eligible for.

Category	Sample $	Category	My $
Desired Mortgage Amount	$150,000	Desired Mortgage Amount	$
Interest Rate	5.50%	Interest Rate	
Annual Income	$72,000	Annual Income	$
Hypothetical Mortgage Payment (Principle & Interest)	$915 per month	Hypothetical Mortgage Payment (Principle & Interest) (Pick a monthly payment that your household would be comfortable with)	$
+ Hypothetical Property Taxes	$100 per month	+ Hypothetical Property Taxes	$
+ Hypothetical Secondary Mortgage	$000	+ Hypothetical Secondary Mortgage	$
+ Hypothetical Heating costs	$50	+ Hypothetical Heating costs	$
+ Hypothetical Condo Fee (50% of it)	$150	+ Hypothetical Condo Fee (50% of it)	$
= Total Monthly Costs divided by Gross Monthly Income (Up to 32% of Your Gross Monthly Income)	$1,215 (of possible $1,920 GDS)	= Total Monthly Costs divided by Gross Monthly Income (Up to 32% of Your Gross Monthly Income)	$
Total Debt Service Ratio (Monthly)	Gross Debt Service amount is $1,215	**Total Debt Service Ratio (Monthly)**	Gross Debt Service amount =
+Monthy Payments and other debts (loans, car, credit cards)	Car +$350 Credit cards + $400 Total = $750	+Monthy Payments and other debts (loans, car, credit cards)	$
= Total Monthly Costs divided by Total Monthly Income	GDS + Debts of $750 = $1,965	= Total Monthly Costs divided by Total Monthly Income	GDS + Debts=TDS
(Up to 40% of Your Gross Monthly Income)	(of possible $2,400 TDS)	(Up to 40% of Your Gross Annual Income	

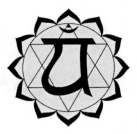

The *Asanas*: Half Spinal Twist & Crescent Moon

Practicing the *asanas* that bend you backwards or elevate your heart over your head opens you to the feelings of trust and love for yourself and family that will continue to motivate your financial mission.

Posture: *Ardha-matsyendra-asana* (Half Spinal Twist)

Ardha means half in Sanskrit. *Matsyendra* translates as King of the Fishes, the name of an ancient yoga master. Because the back is gently twisted, this pose is called the Half Spinal Twist.

- Sit on the floor with legs straight in front of you, then bend your knees to your chest. Slide your left foot under your right leg until it is outside your right hip. Lay the outer part of left leg on the floor. Step the right foot over the left leg so that the right knee points to the ceiling.

- Twist and press the right hand against the floor just behind your right buttock, place upper left arm close to the knee on the outside right thigh.

- Firmly press the inner right foot against the floor. Lean back slightly with the upper torso back slightly .

- By turning your head to the right you can complete the twist of your torso. Turning your head to the left counters the twist.

- Reverse leg, arm and spine positions, and repeat pose.

Ardha-matsyendra-asana (Half Spinal Twist)

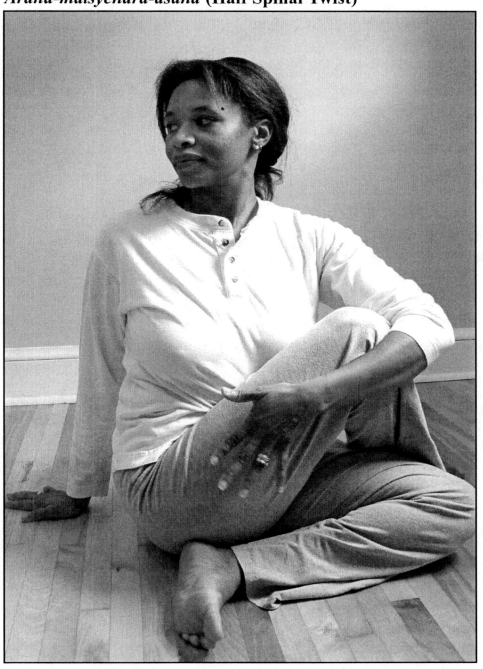

Posture: *Ardha Chandrasana* (Crescent Moon)

The Sanskrit word *Ardha* means half or crescent and *Chandra* means moon.

- Put fingertips or palms on floor next to feet.

- Take a large step back with the right leg, arching your torso and head.

- Lift your hands above your head, reaching for the ceiling with palms together, thumbs crossed and index fingers pointing straight up.

- Beginning with the toes of your right foot, arch all the way through the leg, torso, and arms, finishing with the fingertips. If this is too hard, you can keep your knee on the floor and, as you gain strength, begin to straighten the leg until you achieve the full pose.

- Make sure your elbows are locked and that your head is tilted back with eyes focused on the ceiling.

- Switch legs and repeat this pose.

Ardha Chandrasana (Crescent Moon)

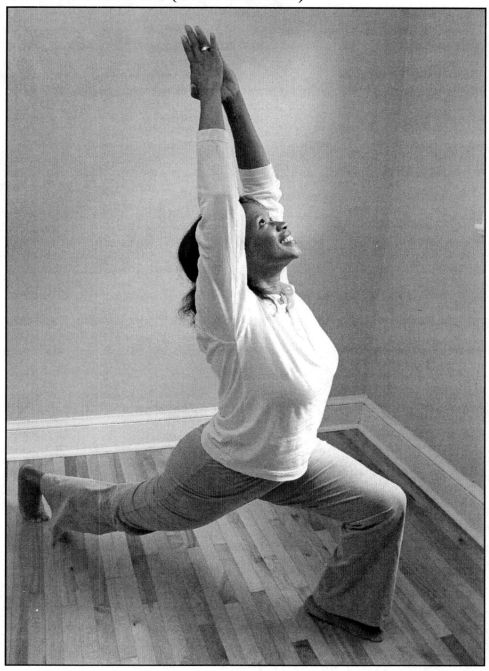

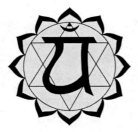

4ᵀᴴ Chakra: Additional Information

·   The gemstones specific to this chakra are rose quartz and jade.

·   The associated essential oils are geranium and rose.

·   Green is the primary colour for this chakra.

·   The sound mantra for meditation is "Yam."

·   The sense associated with this chakra is touch.

·   The chakra is located in the center of the chest.

·   The challenge of "I love" is to honour your ideal of love while maintaining appropriate, caring boundaries.

·   The element associated with this chakra is Air. It energizes the body and feeds the mind. Air permeates all spaces, finding its shape according to its environment. Let your environment shape your financial decisions.

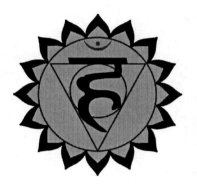

5TH CHAKRA

Vissudha (Throat)
I Communicate
Asanas: Corpse & Wind Release

The fifth chakra in the life wheel is called *Vissudha* (Throat). It is the first of the chakras to align solely with mental and spiritual energy. When this chakra is balanced, you communicate your inner voice to the outside world with clarity, strength and creativity.

Vissudha translates from Sanskrit as "pure" or "purification." The ancient yogis believed that a pure and subtle vibration was the beginning of all creation. Hence, this chakra is associated with the communication of your thoughts and creative impulses. Imbalance in the Throat chakra goes in two directions. If it is too active, others find that you have poor listening skills, typically because you are talking excessively and are unable to take the mental pause to hear their voices. When it is sluggish, you have problems speaking your truth, which manifests as withdrawal, poor boundaries, and the likelihood that, when you finally express yourself, it will be with anger.

Indicators of a balanced Throat chakra include the pleasure you find in singing along to the radio, writing a conversational letter to a friend or the confidence to calmly voice your opinions in any situation. You intuitively understand that a happy life is created by your beliefs and ideas and how successfully you translate them into action. You know that communication is both expression (whether voice, movement or visual art) and listening. When you give a panhandler a dollar, you also share a heart-felt greeting. You are sharing your abundance. Just as you hope the universe will share its abundance with you.

In the Christian ethos the "Adam's apple" comes from the idea that a piece of the forbidden apple stuck in Adam's throat. This is a perfect symbol of the fear of success, self-imposed limitaions and blocked creative flows that come from an imbalance in the Throat chakra. You find yourself unable to share your struggles with money, even with close friends or family members. You feel shame and guilt. Rather than admit the truth of your financial situation, you go out for a meal you can ill afford, or buy an expensive birthday gift for a co-worker instead of simply writing them a card. It may also show up in your inability to sit down with your partner and have that hard talk about shared debts and risky spending habits.

The Conversation

It was well into the dog days of summer and Jane and her daughter Lily hadn't yet taken advantage of the beautiful warm days. The life of a single working mom can be busy, frustrating and lonely. Jane knew she hadn't spent enough time with her daughter. She decided to take a moment and create a little joy.

She booked a day at the cottage, consciously deciding that it wouldn't matter what kind of weather Mother Nature brought on. She and Lily were going to play.

They had a great Saturday at the cottage, surprising Jane, as Lily had been a little high maintenance over the last six months. She had been moody and less than polite. That day it seemed like the sullen, rude stranger had been replaced by the calm, thoughtful, respectful, and beautiful daughter that Jane had given birth to. Yahoo! Her baby was back! At least for a little while, and Jane decided to enjoy it.

A few days later, Lily called Jane to her "office." This is the place where Lily takes advantage of MSN, catalogues her music, burns CDs, and hopefully, does her homework. She had decided to interrupt her busy day, "Maahhmmm! I have to show you something."

Jane walked in to hear Lily announce, "Listen to this. I'm going to play it at your funeral." Silence. Dead silence. No pun intended. Lilly hit play on her music list and it was a song they both knew and loved. Jane didn't know where this was going and I am sure you can appreciate that it was tough to process this scenario. Her funeral? Jane had attended her grandaunt and great grandmother's funerals, but that was years ago.

They listened to the first four lines. Jane looked at Lily and saw so much love and appreciation for their life together. They began to sing louder and louder in harmony. Mother and daughter were communicating on a level that was original, intimate and immense.

Jane and Lily's shared moment reinforces my belief that life is to be savoured. You can't predict when your time will come. But, for my children, I will plan. I could not forgive myself if I did not prepare for the time when they will have to choose a song to commemorate my passing and celebrate my life. As much as we hate to think about it, there comes a day when our last breath is exhaled. Use some of your breaths right now to plan for that time and make it easer for the people you love.

The Money: Wills and Family

Love always involves responsibility.

William Barclay

Develop a plan to protect your family's assets.

In principle, humans know what to expect at the end of a life journey.

Knowing that, we can take the time to clarify our desires using some basic estate principles. Ensure that your wishes are carried out without guesswork at a difficult time.

In the next fifty years, an estimated $40 trillion dollars in wealth transfers will take place in North America. Less than 50% of the population has a will. Many clients who do not have a will tend to ask this one question, "Am I rich enough to need a will?" My answer is, "A will is for anyone who has someone with something to lose when you die."

If your estate is simple, there are boxed wills, like boxed divorces, that you can purchase from office supply stores for under $20. Please book an appointment with a professional lawyer to review it. Communication needs to be very clear when dealing with financial and legal matters. Particularly with matters of the heart.

Have *the* conversation with the parties involved so that they are not surprised when the will is disbursed. The love you feel for them now can be expressed in planning for the time when you can't be there to support them.

Remember that your estate can still be contested if the people in your life feel they are obliged to more than you have left them.

Note that laws interpreting the terms and terminology used in your will may be different between provinces.

Good estate planning begins with

· Documenting your wishes.

· Establishing a strategy to "gift" your assets to family members, charities, and other organizations.

· Choosing an emotionally strong Executor. Will they help with the funeral arrangements?

· Deciding who will take care of the kids. Plan for a guardian.

Think about who you want to provide for. Considerations include your spouse/common law partner, ex-spouse, children and stepchildren, extended family, friends, business partners, coworkers and charities.

Some Common Questions

1. What is a guardian?

A guardian is the person you appoint in your will to raise your minor children. If no guardian is named in your will, the courts will select a guardian on your behalf. Hopefully, you will have had a discussion about your wishes with the person(s) you designate as your guardian. Make sure that they will have sufficient funds for your children's expenses and also ensure that your children's inheritance is protected in the event the guardian goes "bad."

2. What is a Power of Attorney and why would I require one?

It is now becoming common practice to have a Power of Attorney for Property prepared at the same time you have a will prepared. This means that you can appoint someone to manage your financial affairs in the event that you are unable to. You may also appoint someone to make decisions on your behalf regarding your personal care and consent to treatment if you are unable to do so. This is known as the Power of Attorney for Personal Care. Both Powers of Attorney may be revoked at any time as long as you have the requisite mental capacity.

3. What is a "living will"?

"Living will" is a term commonly used to describe a document that expresses an individual's desires and directives regarding medical treatment when that individual is in a terminal state. Often the living will prohibits life-support systems that may prolong life artificially.

4. What is a spouse?

There is a common misconception that if a couple lives together for a long enough period of time they will acquire the same rights as a married spouse under the law.

- Under the Income Tax Act, a spouse is defined as married or not married but having cohabited for one year.

- Under the Succession Law Reform Act, which relates to distribution of property when there is no will, spouse is defined as married only.

- Under the Family Law Act Parts I and II, you must be married in order to have the right to equalize net family property and the right to possession of the matrimonial home.
- Part III of the Family Law Act relating to the right for support defines a spouse as married or having cohabited for three years or in a relationship of some permanence if they have a child.

If a common law spouse dies without a will, the remaining common law spouse is not entitled to share in the property of the deceased (they may have a claim for support under certain circumstances). If the deceased spouse dies without a will and is still legally married without having completed a separation agreement dealing with these issues, the person to whom they are legally married when they pass away would be entitled to the first $200,000 of the estate with the balance divided among the married spouse and children.

As a rule of thumb, make sure you have an up-to-date will, a binding cohabitation agreement, a pre-nuptial contract, and/or a separation agreement.

Upon your death, the government will take a large portion of your estate. Fill out the worksheets below to see how taxes will impact the inheritance you leave to your family. A tax accountant or estate specialist lawyer can help to minimize the amount that the government claims, leaving more for your loved ones.

CATEGORY	CURRENT VALUE
ASSETS:	
Cash in Savings Accounts	
Cash in Checking Accounts	
Cash on Hand	
Money Market Accounts	
Money Owed to Me	
Cash Value of Life Insurance	
Savings Bonds (Current Value)	
Stocks	
Bonds	
Mutual Funds	
Vested Value of Stock Options	
Other Investments	
Registered Retirement Savings Plans	

CATEGORY	CURRENT VALUE
Registered Retirement Income Fund	
Other Retirement Plans	
Market Value of Your Home	
Market Value of Other Real Estate	
Blue Book Value of Cars/Trucks	
Boats, Planes, Other Vehicles	
Jewelry	
Collectibles	
Furnishings and Other Personal Property	
Other	
TOTAL ASSETS	
LIABILITIES:	
Mortgages	
Car Loans	
Bank Loans	
Student Loans	
Home Equity Loans	
Other Loans	
Credit Card Balances	
Real Estate Taxes Owed	
Income Taxes Owed	
Other Taxes Owed	
Other Debts	
TOTAL LIABILITIES	
NET WORTH (TOTAL ASSETS MINUS TOTAL LIABILITIES)	

Worksheet: Determining Estate Taxes

Formula	Example	Your Numbers
Your Gross Assets	Three million	
Minus-Your Debts	- $100,000	
Minus-Transfers to your spouse	- $500,000	
Minus-Credit exemption	- $1,500,000	
= Your taxable estate	= $900,000	
X Multiply tax rate	@ 45%	
= Estate tax	= about $450,000	

Use the information you've just charted to determine the taxes on your estate.

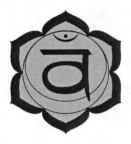

The *Asanas*: Corpse Pose & Wind Release Pose

These *asanas* encourage acceptance and the act of letting go. They will help you develop the willingness for actions that ensure those you love are looked after once you leave the body behind.

Posture: *Shava-asana* (Corpse)

The Sanskrit word *shava* means corpse. It is also referred to as the *Yoga Nidra*, which is the deep state of relaxation that this posture creates.

- Lie on your back with your eyes closed. Relax your body and let your palms gently curl upwards. Breathe normally.

- You can also choose to relax your mind by focusing it on an object or place that you find pleasant and soothing.

Shava-asana (Corpse)

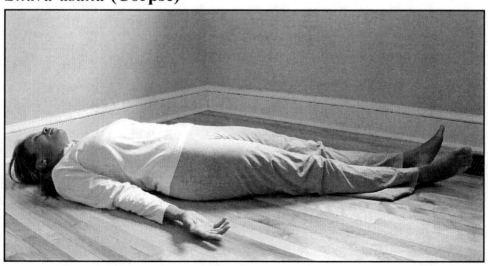

Posture: *Pavana-mukta-asana* (Wind Release)

The Sanskrit word *pavana* means air or wind, and *mukta* means freedom or release. This posture is aptly named, as it helps release uncomfortable abdominal gases.

- Sit on the floor and stretch your legs out in front of you.
- Rest your hands on the floor beside your hips.
- Keep your torso straight and make sure your chin is parallel to the floor.
- Stretch your toes out while keeping your heels to the ground.
- Bend your right leg, bringing the knee close into the chest.
- Put your right hand on your bent right knee.
- Lift the knee toward the right shoulder.
- Place right hand on the inside of the right foot and reach for the right heel. Try and bring the knee as close to your right shoulder as possible.
- Breathe deeply.
- Switch leg and arm, and repeat posture.

Pavana-mukta-asana (Wind Release)

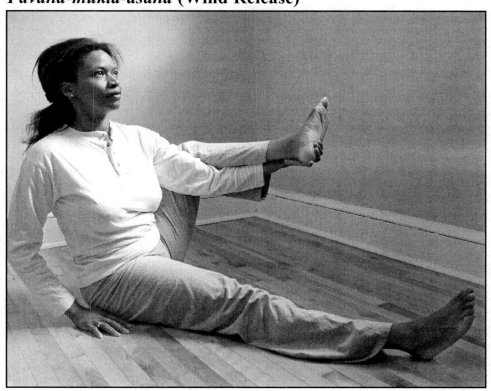

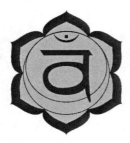

5ᵀᴴ Chakra: Additional Information

- The gemstone specific to this region is turquoise.

- The associated essential oils are myrrh and spearmint.

- Blue is the primary colour for this chakra.

- The sound mantra for meditation is "*Ham.*"

- The sense associated with this chakra is hearing.

- The chakra is located at the center of the throat and connects to the entire nervous system.

- The challenge of "I communicate" comes from the responsibility to shape and maintain healthy relationships.

- The element associated with this chakra is *Akasa* (ether), the basic element that forms earth, fire, water and air. It is considered the medium of sound and communication, both internal and external. It carries the inner voice that supports financial sanity.

6TH CHAKRA

Ajna (Brow or Third Eye)
I Know
Asanas (positions): Warrior Two & Tree

The sixth chakra in the life wheel is the *Ajna* (Brow) chakra. It is the site of imagination and perception (also known as the Third Eye). Balance in the *Ajna* chakra gives you the ability to make the positive visualizations that attract a healthy, happy and manageable life.

The *Ajna* chakra (which directly translates as "command") controls your ability to make your hopes and dreams a reality. When it is unbalanced you have difficulty visualizing where you want your life to lead and how you will get there. If this chakra is overactive it may manifest as frantic attempts to manipulate your environment and an inability to concentrate; you find yourself with a million ideas but lack the focus to make even one of them a reality. Conversely, an under-active *Ajna* chakra prevents you from using anything but your most concrete mental processes. You are unable to predict the likely results of your actions, whether good or bad.

This energy point is also the place where your perception of the material world blends with your spiritual life. It doesn't matter if you worship within a formal spiritual program or have a more intuitive sense of a higher power. Balance in this chakra infuses your spirit with a sane attitude toward money, stopping the behaviours that create financial problems for you and your family.

The Conversation

I have a good friend, Maxine, who intuitively understands that life's direction can change. She used to work out too much; now she does just the right amount to stay healthy. She never wore sunscreen because she loved to tan. Now she wears SPF 30. She used to smoke; now she's a proud quitter. Maxine's busy party lifestyle has been reduced to a couple of glasses of wine a week. She's moved from the undemanding relationships of her twenties into marriage, children and caring for her aging parents.

Recently, she attended a four-day company meeting. On the last day of her conference, she was in the hotel gym when she heard a disturbing "pop" in her back. Showered, changed, and looking the part of an unstoppable young businesswoman, she entered the first session of the day and took a seat next to a colleague. She couldn't stop shaking, which her coworker attributed to the aftermath of the open bar at the previous evening's shindig. But Maxine had left the party early just to avoid any chance of "the morning after." She staggered out of the seminar, averting a fall only by clutching the backs of chairs and then using the walls as support until she made it back to her room.

For the next three weeks she slid from wall to chair to door to wall to car to bed. She finally made an appointment with her doctor. He immediately sent her to the hospital for an MRI and CAT scan. "Don't leave the hospital until you have these tests completed!" he firmly instructed her. A few questions and he reluctantly explained that he was looking for a diagnosis on a scale of one to ten, with one being an inflammation in the spine requiring back surgery and ten being Multiple Sclerosis (MS), a debilitating immune disorder.

The test results came in. She had MS. Maxine was only in her mid-thirties, the age at which the first MS exacerbations are often felt.

· Her first thought—what does my future hold?
· Her second thought—will my insurance look after my family and I?
· Answer to the first thought—as good as she believes it can be.
· Answer to the second thought—only if she's currently got insurance and it covers long-term critical illness financial needs.

Consider who you need to protect before it's too late.

The Money: Your Desired Insurance

Someday is not a day of the week.

Denise Brennan-Nelson

Have you had this inner conversation about insurance? "I don't need it. I'm going to live to be a hundred years old without illness." *No one* wants to pay for insurance. But the longer you wait to buy it, the higher your statistical risk category, which can either make you ineligible for insurance or force you to pay very high rates.

When I'm helping my clients arrange their finances, I always ask, "If you are no longer here to pay the mortgage, how will it impact your family?" I also point out that they should consider the "What ifs" of unexpected illness, the need for extended care, and any other curve balls that life might throw at them.

Insurance does not have to be a bad news conversation. You have insurance on you credit cards and line of credit, your car, your home's contents and other possessions, but you don't have insurance for yourself!

There must be a balance between the cost of insurance and your investment savings. Look at insurance both as a way to cover you now and as an investment to cover you in retirement.

Part of the journey towards financial health is insurance—life, mortgage, disability and critical illness.

Insurance 101

Life Insurance

The most cost effective way to get life insurance is through work. The younger and healthier you are, the lower the cost of your premiums. If you are single and can afford it, insure yourself for ten times your annual salary. If something happens to you, the insurance proceeds can be invested and you (or your dependants) can live off the investments. If you are part of a couple, then a good rule of thumb is to add up all your combined debts and add an additional $100,000 to $250,000, depending on what you can afford.

There are two main types of life insurance.

Term insurance covers you for a specific amount of time and can be renewed (at a higher cost).

Permanent insurance covers you for your life-time and includes an investment portion.

Disability Insurance

Disability insurance is designed to protect you from the loss of an asset far more valuable than your home or your car; your potential lifetime income. The odds that a disability may impact on your work life are probably higher than you imagine.

Again, the most cost effective way to get this is through your work plan. It is better if *you* make the actual payments, because if your employer pays for the insurance the income you receive from it becomes taxable. You should be covered for about 70% of your gross income. If you are not covered twenty-four hours a day, seven days a week through your work plan, you might want to look at getting another policy to cover you outside of work. Also, check to see if you are covered under your own occupation or any occupation, as this will affect you in the event of a permanent disability.

Chances of becoming disabled for 3 months or longer before age 65*

Percentage	58%	54%	50%	48%	40%	30%	23%
Age	25	30	35	40	45	50	55

* Derived from 1985 Commissioners Individual Disability Table A.

Critical Illness Insurance

More and more people are living through critical illnesses like cancer, stroke, and heart disease. There are many costs beyond loss of income associated with critical illness, such as medical supplies, professional care-givers, and accessibility alterations to the home. Typically, lack of proper insurance means drawing on your RRSPs to cover costs. On average this will push your retirement plans back ten years.

Health and Dental Insurance

If you have this through work, check to see if you will be covered after retirement, as many corporations have stopped insuring their retirees. If you have doubts, it is better to get private extended health and dental insurance when you are younger and healthier. Depending on your health, you may not be able to find coverage when you are older.

Who Will You Protect?

Take a few minutes to answer the questions below; they will help put your insurance needs in perspective.

You may also find it helpful to create a small scrapbook, using photographs of yourself and your family and assign symbols for the type of protection you will give them (e.g. your parents: help with long-term care; yourself: income to preserve your standard of living in case of a sudden or long-term illness).

My current monthly budget requires: $ _____
(Use budget from first chapter.)

In the event of long-term illness and mental or physical trauma, do I have adequate insurance to meet my budget needs? **Yes**_____ **No** _____

In the event of long-term illness and mental or physical trauma, do I have adequate insurance to cover the costs of modifying my home to accommodate my needs? **Yes**_____ **No** _____

In the event of long-term illness and mental or physical trauma, do I have adequate insurance to cover the costs that future care needs may incur? **Yes**_____ **No** _____

Who, in the event of my death, long-term illness or traumatic accident, do I want to provide for financially?

_____

_____

_____

_____

Do I have adequate insurance to ensure that I am not a financial burden to these people in the event of my death, long-term illness or traumatic accident? **Yes_____ No _____**

Do I have adequate insurance to provide for the needs of my family in the event of my death, long-term illness or traumatic accident? **Yes_____ No _____**

If you replied no to most of these questions, it is time to start making appointments with insurance agents.

First, prioritize your insurance needs according to your circumstances. For example, if you are a single parent with minor children, you will want to ensure that you have sufficient insurance to meet your children's future living and education costs. You may not be able to afford all the insurance you need immediately, but you can start the process of protecting yourself and the people you love.

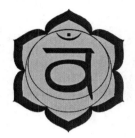

The *Asanas*: Warrior Two & Tree

These *asanas* will give you the stamina needed to look beyond the immediate and decide what your future will be. Envision a secure financial future and the actions involved in reaching it.

Posture: *Virabhadra* (Warrior)

Named after a warrior incarnation of Shiva, this *asana* enables the loving acts of strength that transform us into grateful warriors for those we love (hopefully, this includes ourselves).

- Start from a standing position, arms by your side, and take a large step forward with the right foot.

- Hips are square in front (no twist). Shift the left foot so that the arch of the left foot is in line with the heel of the right foot.

- Leaning into the right leg, ensuring that the knee is not over the toes, inhale the arms straight up and hold this Warrior One position.

- Now, shift the weight slowly and deliberately forward, coming up on the toes of the left foot and leaning forward, lifting the heel toward the ceiling.

- Extend the arms forward and lengthen from the crown of the head along the spine then the leg and let the energy release through the toes.

- Switch forward leg and repeat posture.

Virabhadra (**Warrior**)

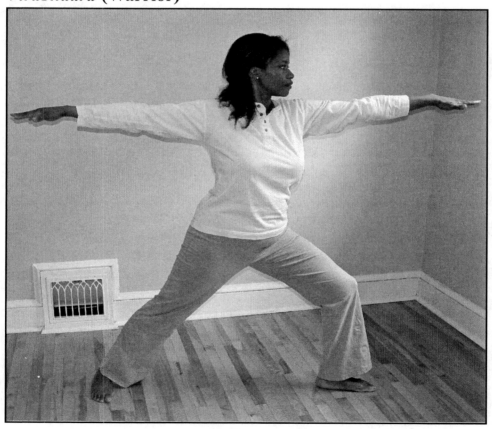

Posture: *Vrksasana* (Tree)

- The tree (*vrksa* in Sanskrit) is symbolic of the hidden self reaching for the sun as it emerges from the earth.
- Begin in the *tadasana*.
- Bring your hands to your waist, and then relax the shoulders.
- Shift your weight to the right foot.
- Lift your knee to the waist. Open the knee out to the side and lift. Take left foot and place above or below the knee.
- Use your core strength to prevent unnecessary pressure on the right knee.
- Focus on an unmoving object and envision that your supporting leg is the strong trunk of a tree.
- Allow the branches (your arms) to grow upward, arms framing the head, and put your palms together.
- Switch leg and repeat posture.

Vrksasana (Tree)

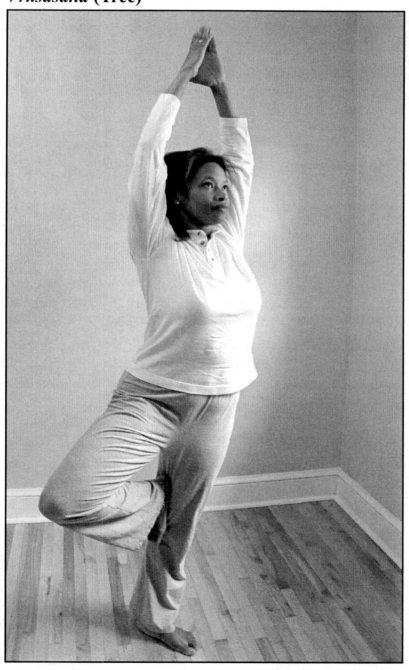

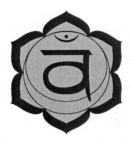

6ᵀᴴ Chakra: Additional Information

·   The gemstone specific to this chakra is amethyst.

·   The associated essential oil is lavender.

·   Indigo is the primary colour for this chakra.

·   The sound mantra for mediation is "Om."

·   The sense associated with this chakra is intuition.

·   The chakra is located just above the eyes, in the center of the brow.

·   The challenge of "I know" lies in translating your creative imaginings and spiritual life into actions in the material world.

·   The element associated with this chakra is Time. Through your imagination you can move through this element in any direction. Use this power to visualize the actions you will take and the rewards you will receive as you move toward financial health.

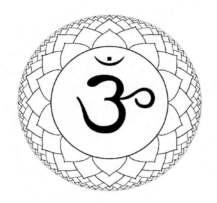

7ᵀᴴ CHAKRA

Sahasrara (Crown)

I Think

Asanas (Positions): Headstand & Plough

The seventh chakra is the Crown or, in Sanskrit, the *Sahasrara*. Balance in this chakra can only be achieved when the other six are in harmony. The underlying sense of connection with life gives you the faith and strength to act from your ethics and values, rather than your fears.

Sahasrara also translates as thousand-fold, an ancient expression for the infinite essence that flows through everything, including you. If your seventh chakra is too active, you live in your head, disconnected from your heart and body. You may believe yourself better than those around you and experience frustration with their inability to recognize your superiority. When this chakra is inactive, you are apathetic and prefer not to think for yourself. In both cases, your lack of connection with a higher power ensures that your relationship with money is problematic.

When the *Sahasrara* is balanced, you are in a position to become a guide and mentor. Share the lessons you have learned on the path to financial freedom. Begin with your family and then expand to your friends and colleagues.

You move from feeling you must always be doing to a state of contentment in simply being. At this point, the journey has become more important than the end result. You no longer race around worrying about how to make money. You may not be a millionaire, but you have control over your finances and are comfortable. Because you are aware, happy, and secure, you are in a position to be of service.

The Conversation

At only twelve years of age Lily created her own business. She decided she'd seen enough of mom's questionable employment strategies; she opened her own spa and babysitting service. She found a partner and trained a third girlfriend to provide manicures and pedicures.

Jane had to ask her, "Why are you doing this?" Lily's answer? "Because mom, I've seen you work so hard and you really need some pampering." Did Jane cry? Yes. You truly never know what you've taught your children until they show you.

Lily, with her love for children, her babysitter certification and the book on babysitting she had personally created, decided to take on the childcare, plus the head and neck massages while also managing the business promotion. She soon had her mobile spa ready to go, complete with the email address, flyers and magnetic business cards.

Jane helped Lily distribute her flyers around the neighborhood, awed by her daughter's initiative. It did not stop there. She had her 30-second "unique sales proposition" memorized and ready to go at Mom's and Stepdad's networking associations. Was Jane a proud mom? Absolutely. She knew adults who could not deliver the process that Lily did.

While Lily was building her empire, Jane decided to share some of her hard-won knowledge with her daughter. She booked an appointment for Lily with her own financial advisor, so that they could seriously discuss what Lily's savings and investment options might be. Lily's friends wondered what her mom was up to. Jane wasn't planning on dictating how Lily could spend her earnings, she simply hoped that making the information available might help Lily avoid some of the pain and stress that circumstances, combined with poor financial decisions, often bring in later life.

It's never too early—or too late—to be fiscally proactive. Once you've found the balance between financial risk and reward, it is your responsibility to share your experience and knowledge. An enlightened individual finds joy by helping others succeed.

The Money: A Step Beyond

The greatest good you can do for another is not just to share your riches but to reveal to him his own.

Benjamin Disraeli

In the spirit of sharing, Fraser Smith teaches a technique that converts the largest debt of a Canadian's lifetime (the mortgage) into "good" debt—the kind that is tax-deductible and generates annual refunds from the tax department.

The strategy, called the *Smith Manoeuvre*, is a simple and legal strategy based on Canada Revenue laws that make the interest on a mortgage payment tax deductible.

In Canada, any interest you pay on money that is borrowed for investing is tax deductible. You simply take any money you have in stocks, GIC's, bonds, etc., pay off your mortgage and then borrow the money against your equity to buy your investments back.

This might sound scary, but financially savvy Canadians have been doing it for a long time. Another advantage is that you can start building your retirement investments immediately, rather than waiting till you've paid off your mortgage. If you've got 30% equity built up in your mortgage, the *Smith Manouevre* will work for you. You can calculate just how much more quickly you can pay off your mortgage at www.smithman.net.

Excerpted from *The Smith Manoeuver*, reproduced with permission from the author.

THERE'S AN ELEPHANT HIDING IN YOUR HOUSE

Statistics Canada advises that there are approximately 3.5 million families who own a home with a mortgage. The total mortgage debt that is currently being serviced by these families is about 500 billion dollars. The banks and other lenders are collecting a reasonable market-driven interest rate from the homeowners. Unlike Americans, Canadians are unable to claim their mortgage interest as a tax deduction.

Those 500 billion dollars has been borrowed and spent by Canadians to purchase their homes. The money has been used. But there is a very large opportunity hidden in plain sight. It is that same 500 billion dollars. Because of Canadian tax rules regarding the deductibility of interest, that money can be used a second time. 500 billion of non-deductible house mortgages can and should be converted into 500 billion in tax-deductible investment loans. We have found the elephant. It is your house mortgage.

The investment industry, working with both the willing assistance of the lending industry and the financial planning industry, should embark now on a mission to teach the population about the benefits of converting their mortgage loans (bad debt) to investment loans (good debt). If this mortgage debt were to be converted as suggested, the process would release 500 billion dollars into the economy to purchase investments for the homeowners. This rather simple act of debt conversion makes the interest expense tax deductible for the homeowner. The process costs next to nothing to implement and all the players benefit, especially those families converting their debt from the bad kind to the good kind.

More important than the tax refunds is the fact that the homeowners will begin gathering assets **now** as opposed to after they have spent many years trying to pay off the mortgage. Holding constant a debt already taken (the mortgage) in order to accumulate investments early in life, has a demonstrably superior financial outcome compared to the process most Canadians currently follow—pay off the mortgage, then begin an investment program.

Benefits for the Homeowner

1. *Debt will not increase.* Instead, it will remain constant until conversion has been completed. This is a debt conversion strategy, not a leveraging strategy.

2. The rate of interest will be low (prime or better) since the house is the security for the investment credit line.

3. Any reduction of the first mortgage is borrowed back and used to purchase investments—starting immediately.

4. The interest expense on the investment credit line will generate a tax deduction. The tax deduction will produce a tax refund cheque.

5. The tax refund cheque each year will be used to pay the mortgage down even faster. The amount paid down against the mortgage will be immediately re-borrowed and invested.

6. The tax refunds will get larger each year as conversion progresses.

7. The investment portfolio will compound its value over the years ahead.

8. The investments will be free and clear because the house is the security for the investment loan, not the investments themselves.

9. Since the investment portfolio is free and clear, there can be no margin call.

10. The process is reversible. Since the investments are free and clear they will be available in times of trouble to protect the home, the homeowner and the lender.

11. The homeowner will make the choice to invest in stocks, bonds, mutual funds, investment real estate, his own business, or someone else's business. The interest expense will be tax deductible.

12. The investor will automatically be enjoying the benefits that accrue to those who invest regularly and often, starting now.

13. The length of time to complete the conversion is easy to calculate and will vary from family to family, but the strategy *always* reduces the income tax bill. Assuming this "found" money is wisely utilized to make incremental payments against the mortgage, it can also be said that the strategy always reduces the length of the mortgage.

14. The projected investment returns are subject to the usual market risks. Risks are reduced by the long time horizons related to mortgages. Responsible professionals will encourage homeowners to practice asset diversification, to purchase quality investments, to invest regularly and often, to seek professional assistance, and to suppress greed.

Is there a Downside?

1. The proposition put forward requires that the homeowner understands the important difference between the non-deductible debt of their house mortgage and the deductible debt of an investment loan. With this understanding, most will appreciate the advantage of suspending their desire to get to zero debt in order to allow their investment portfolio to accumulate during the conversion process. For some, it will be impossible to live with debt of any kind, good or bad.

2. When the conversion is completed, the homeowner may wish to resume their course to zero debt by starting to make payments on the new deductible investment loan.

   It can be shown mathematically that they will be financially better off to leave the debt in place, paying interest only, once the interest has been made deductible. If this is done, they will receive ongoing tax refund cheques *for the rest of their life*. Moreover, their cash flow can be used to continue to increase their investments rather than being used to pay off a loan they have worked so hard to convert to the deductible variety. Ultimately, that decision is theirs to make. Some people are so debt averse they will do whatever it takes to get to zero debt—even if it means fewer assets and lower income.

If you do decide to take advantage of the tax laws and your mortgage equity, make sure that you find a financial advisor who is experienced in using the *Smith Manoeuvre*. This is important, as many Canadian banks and credit unions have started issuing re-advancable mortgages, but are unclear on their application. You can visit Fraser Smith's website at www.smithman.net for further information.

There's An Elephant Hiding in your House *has been reprinted from* The Smith Manoeuver (2006) *with the kind permission of Fraser Smith.*

A Journal for Financial Health

I find it helpful to keep a financial journal. I suggest that you take the time to create and maintain one as well. Take five to ten minutes each day to record your financial successes and slips. Write down how your daily choices help or hinder your life goals. Include your dreams and early morning musings. Look at the people in your life, and think about who needs your help and what form that help might take. Now that you are assuming financial control, it's time to "be."

Sample Journal Page

Date: January 1

Quote of the Day: *Real generosity toward the future lies in giving all to the present* (Albert Camus)

The day I got *Yoga For Your Personal Finances* I decided to:

Cut back by one coffee a day and go from an extra large to a large coffee—I'll save $3 every work day!

Start looking at travel brochures and figure out how much I'll need to save for my vacation (no credit card holiday *this* year).

Talk to my immediate family and suggest that, instead of buying birthday and Christmas presents for the adults, we open RESP accounts for the kids and make an annual contribution, instead of buying gifts that we don't need.

Start a spaghetti and wine Saturday twice a month—I'll invite friends over, make some garlic bread, spaghetti, a big salad, and tell them to bring whatever they want to drink... way more fun than mediocre restaurant food and I'll still save money. Maybe we'll even play games—Scrabble, penny poker, Cranium, etc.

Sarah's having a hard time. I'll give her a call and see if she wants to come for a walk and have the breakfast special at our favourite diner next Saturday morning.

I'm going to start asking my friends and colleagues about their financial advisors with the goal of finding someone I feel comfortable planning my financial future with.

Date:

Quote of the Day:

A month after reading *Yoga for Your Personal Finances*, here are some of the changes that I've made:

A month after reading *Yoga for Your Personal Finances*, when I think about my finances I feel:

A month after reading *Yoga for Your Personal Finances*, here are some of the changes that I'm looking forward to making:

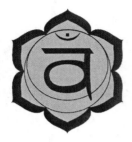

The *Asanas*: Head Stand & Plough

Both of these *asanas* are designed to promote alignment in the brain, activating your seventh chakra. Bear in mind that they are difficult postures and be careful not to push yourself past your comfort zone.

Posture: *Salamba Sirshasana* (Head Stand)

Combining *Salamba* (with support) and *Sirsa* (head), the Sanskrit translation is a reminder of the importance of the care you should take while in this posture.

- Kneel on the floor. Entwine your fingers and place your forearms on a floor mat with elbows at shoulder width. Then set the top of your head on the floor. (Beginners to this pose should press the bases of palms together and place the back of the head against the clasped hands. You may want to use the walls in a room-corner to help you balance.)

- Lift knees from the floor and move feet close to elbows with the heels off the floor. Lift the inverted Vee formed by the tops of your thighs.

- Keep your torso straight through the incline.

- Lift both feet from the floor at the same time and hold the position.

Salamba Sirshasana (Head Stand)

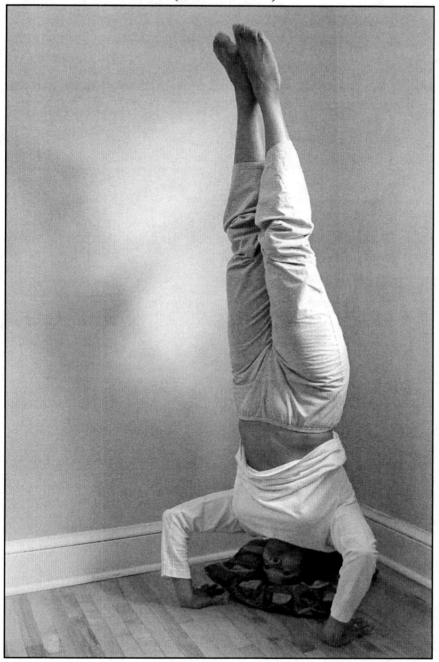

Posture: *Hala-asana* (Plough)

The Sanskrit word *Hala* refers to the traditional plough that is drawn by a horse or oxen. When performing this posture, your body resembles a plough.

- Begin this pose on your back in the *sadasana*.

- Lift legs straight up, pressing the heel to the ceiling.

- Press the shoulders into the floor.

- With hands on the lower back, lift the hips and take the legs straight up.

- From the shoulder stand, gently lower toes over the head and to the ground.

Hala-asana (**Plough**)

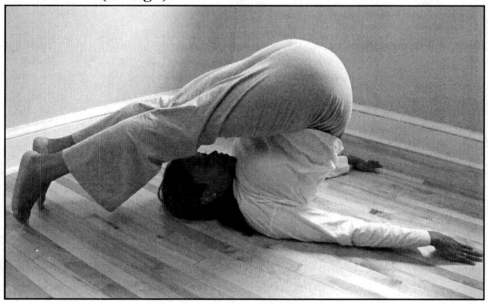

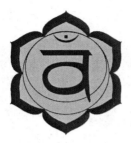

7ᵀᴴ Chakra Additional Information

·   The gemstone specific to this region is diamond.

·   The associated essential oils are jasmine and frankincense.

·   Violet is the primary colour for this chakra.

·   The sound mantra for meditation is absolute silence.

·   All senses are associated with this chakra.

·   The Crown is located on the top of the skull.

·   The challenge of "I think" is to retain faith in the larger pattern of life that is too vast for any individual to comprehend.

·   The element associated with this chakra is cosmic energy. Considered the wellspring of potential, thought originates in this element. Your thoughts shape all aspects of your life, including your finances.

APPENDIX I

More About Yoga

The full practice of yoga is about far more than the *asanas* (poses). It is about a life that is ethical and spiritual. It teaches you awareness and action, as opposed to the unconscious reactions that do so much damage in your life. It's about acting from a place of honour, no matter what anyone else is doing. It's about facing your financial realities and taking concrete, balanced action, instead of letting your unwillingness to do so lure you into get-rich-quick schemes that never work.

Yoga is an inter-related set of eight disciplines.

1. The *Yamas* are five behaviour patterns that enhance the relationship of the individual with the outside world. Designed to restrain the lower nature, they should be practiced in thought, word and deed.

    Ahimsa or non-violence.

    Satyam or truthfulness.

    Brahmacharya or moderation (control of the senses).

    Asteya or non-stealing.

    Aparigraha or non-covetousness (lack of greed).

2. The *Niyamas* (laws) are personal and intimate rules for the internal self.

    Saucha or purity of the mind and body.

Santosha or contentment.

Tapas or austerity.

Swadhyaya or study of the sacred texts.

Ishwara Pranidhana or awareness of, and surrender to, a divine presence.

3. *Asana* means staying or abiding. In the Western culture *asanas* are called poses and are what most people think of when the word yoga comes up. Practice of the *asansas* brings a corresponding mental balance between the body and the mind, strengthening and healing the physical body. EEG studies of individuals performing *asanas* show a calming effect on the brain.

4. *Pranayama* is control of the breath. It goes hand in hand with the *asanas*. It is a form of purification and self-discipline that works to calm the mind and body.

5. *Pratyahara* means drawing back or retreat. It is a withdrawal from the sensual world that quiets the mind. It implies the loss of any attachment to external objects.

6. *Dharana* is concentration. It is a meditation that focuses the attention in one direction or on one object. It is a way to prevent the mind from dissipating its energy in too many directions.

7. *Dhyana* means perfect contemplation. It is a meditation of pure thought that seeks the truth of the object being focused upon.

8. *Samadhi* (to bring together) is the last step. It is a state where mind and body are transcended and you experience a sense of oneness with all around you.

APPENDIX II
Make Your Time Your Own–21 Days in 7 Days

Some of the impediments to your financial health originate in time management. Do you eat out or buy expensive, ready-made meals instead of cooking for yourself because you lack the time to shop and prepare meals? Do you take a taxi (or drive and pay parking fees) because you haven't got the time to walk a few blocks? Do you find that you never have enough time and compensate by "treating" yourself to luxuries that you can ill-afford?

You can really help yourself by writing down what you do all week and the time you spend on each activity. As you track how you spend your time, you can learn to cut out things like television (a big time waster), non-productive talk at work, procrastination in all its many forms, and the other things that waste your time and contribute to your emotional and financial stress.

I suggest you break up each of your 24-hour days into three segments, based on the time you have before work, the time you spend at work and the time between the end of the workday and bedtime. Repeat this schedule for the next six days to create your 21 "days" in a week.

The idea is to maximize your mornings and evenings by getting to sleep early so you can wake up early. Try to leave work on time so you have time in the evenings.

Make sure you make appointments during your 21-day week for the things that are important to you such as: going out with friends, reading, movies, a massage, fooling around, and, of course, your yoga time. Try to take advantage of the free events that your community offers—a concert, a walk in the park, lectures at the library and so forth. You will not only help your budget, but you will also find that stepping outside of your normal routine gives you mini-vacations that refresh the spirit.

Day One begins when your head leaves the pillow until your hand turns the doorknob as you enter work.

Day Two begins when you touch the doorknob upon arriving at work, and ends when you touch the doorknob as you leave work.

Day Three begins the moment you leave work, and finishes when your head hits the pillow.

Sample "Day"

Day One 5 am to 8:55 am	Day Two 9:00 am to 5:25 pm	Day Three 5:30 pm to 9 pm
Read newspaper. Yoga. Walk. Make breakfast & lunch. Answer emails.	Arrive at office. Prioritize mandatory/ important tasks. Lunch at restaurant with co-workers. Meeting with clients. Sales reports.	Write birthday card. Grocery list. Dinner. Homework. Clean up. Phone friend. Read novel. Go to bed.

Your 21 Day Week

Monday

Day One	Day Two	Day Three

Tuesday

Day One	Day Two	Day Three

Wednesday

Day One	Day Two	Day Three

Thursday

Day One	Day Two	Day Three

Friday

Day One	Day Two	Day Three

Saturday

Day One	Day Two	Day Three

Sunday

Day One	Day Two	Day Three

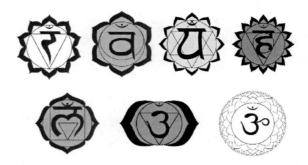

CONCLUSION

Back at the lakeshore, there is squawking coming from the falcon's nest. It is time for the young nestlings to learn how to fly. They are reluctant, naturally afraid of leaving the only environment they have ever known. The parent falcons nudge them with their beaks, pushing them against the edge. You hold your breath and watch, hoping that mom and dad are right and the chicks are ready to take flight. The boldest fledgling begins to flap its wings and suddenly makes the leap of faith. For a moment it falls, then the air catches it and the bird is aloft—only for a few seconds, until it makes an awkward landing at a nearby tree. But with each short flight it improves. Soon it will be able to soar for hours, floating above the land on sun-warmed air currents.

I hope that you are feeling ready to make the leap of faith toward financial health. You began when you decided to pick up this book. Every time you practice the *asanas,* you bring balance to the energy flow of your chakras, giving you the strength and calm needed to do the work suggested here. Each worksheet you filled out has made you more conscious of your financial health. You now have goals and guidelines, which, if you follow them, will give you a healthy and manageable relationship with your money.

Namaste,
Jacqueline

SOURCES

Books Referenced

Bell, Andrew, *Money Management All-in-One Desk Reference for Canadians for Dummies*, John Wiley & Sons Canada Limited, 2003.

Belling, Noa, *Yoga Handbook*, New Holland Publishers Limited, 2003.

Rooman, Lily, *All About Chakras: Knowing and Activating the Body's Energy Centres*, Astrolog Publishing, 2002.

Smith, Fraser, *The Smith Manoeuvre*, Trafford Publishing, 2006.

Websites Referenced

www.santosha.com

www.yogajournal.com

www.webspirit.com

Professional Expertise

Lisa Hyman, Financial Advisor
Asset Money Management
Armstrong & Quaile and associates
www.am-m.ca

Deborah O'Connor, Lawyer
Dust Evans Lawyers/Advocates

ACKNOWLEDGMENTS

Many people helped to make this book a reality. I'm grateful for their support.

I want to thank my mother, Janet, and my grandmother, Monica, who raised their children to believe that they are strong enough to accomplish anything they put their minds to.

My amazing daughter, Merrique, and my encouraging and loving husband, Michael Kelly, were infinitely gracious as the dining room table disappeared under progressive book drafts. I promise them that all the take-out menus are going right into the recycling bin. They also pitched in by critiquing my initial drafts.

When I faltered, my brother, Jason, and sister, Jennifer, reminded me that, even if I am the suit-wearing member of the family, I also share their creative lineage.

For their loving support, I thank Anne-Marie and Siobhan. Marcy Berg of Summit Mortgage Services welcomed me into the next phase of my mortgage career..

And, from inception to publishing, this book was nursed along by *The Non-Dicloure$*—five women who could rule the world!

Finally, I want to acknowledge Book Coach Press for providing the coaching, editorial, and design expertise to make my dream of *Yoga for Your Personal Finances* come true.

ABOUT THE AUTHOR

Jacqueline Richards blends practical financial advice with her personal experience of yoga's mental and physical benefits. She is an accredited mortgage professional with almost twenty years experience in customer service and project management. She took up yoga eight years ago. At the time she was opening a major hotel from the ground up and working fourteen hours a day. She credits her daily yoga sessions with saving her sanity!

Jacqueline teaches Hatha yoga because she wants to share the benefits she found through practicing the *asanas* (postures) and *pranayamas* (breath exercises). The questions students asked when they realized Jacqueline's dual roles of mortgage consultant and yoga instructor inspired *Yoga For Your Personal Finances*. She believes that the principles of balance and flow so fundamental to yoga also apply to money management.

The oldest daughter of globe-trotting parents and a veteran of multiple moves, she treasures the warmth and stability of the home she shares with daughter Merrique and husband Michael. Jacqueline loves books and music, and, under protest, submits to her daughter's ongoing efforts to create the perfect hairstyle for both yoga and banking.

Jacqueline is a firm believer in women in business. She participated in the Prime Minister's Task Force on Female Entrepreneurs, was on the executive of the National Capital Branch of Canadian Women in Communication and is currently chair of the Eastern Ottawa Chamber of Commerce. She is past president of Business Network International (Capital Chapter) and a facilitator with Women Moving Forward (Nepean Chapter).

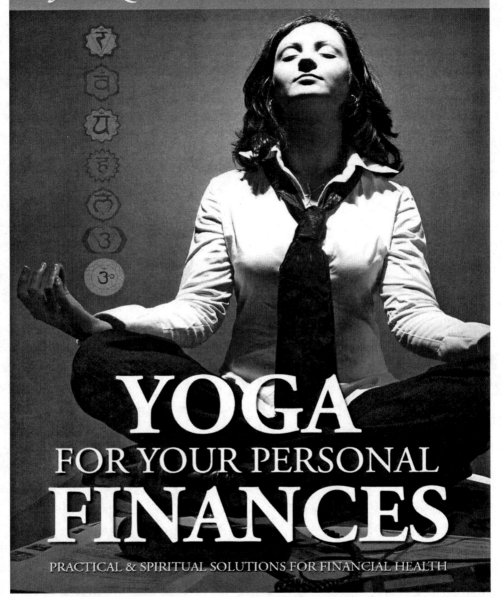

JACQUELINE RICHARDS

YOGA
FOR YOUR PERSONAL
FINANCES

PRACTICAL & SPIRITUAL SOLUTIONS FOR FINANCIAL HEALTH